Dr. Gérard Pacaud

Homeopathy encyclopedia

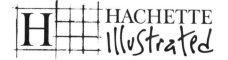

First published by Marabout, an imprint of Hachette-Livre, 43 Quai de Grenelle, Paris 75905, Cedex 15, France under the title *Guide de l'Homéopathie*

This edition published 2003 by Hachette Illustrated UK, Octopus Publishing Group, 2–4 Heron Quays, London E14 4JP
English translation © 2003 Octopus Publishing Group.

ISBN: 1-8420-2190-7

The information and recommendations given in this book are not intended to be a substitute for medical advice. Consult your doctor before acting on any recommendations given in this book. The authors and publisher disclaim any liability, loss, injury or damage incurred as a consequence, directly or indirectly, of the use and application of the contents of this book.

Translation supplied by First Edition Translations Ltd, Cambridge, in conjunction with Book Production Consultants plc, Cambridge.

Printed in

Table of contents

Introduction

This guide is, in the broadest sense, a 'vade mecum' for the adventure of life, in which you are both the actor and the narrator. Your main concern is your health and all its inherent uncertainties. You will be well equipped, as the remedies suggested in this book are effective, and will help you to negotiate the potentially chaotic obstacle course of life.

This form of complementary medicine, which is backed by two centuries of experience, is widespread in Asia and North America and throughout Europe.

I have no doubt that this movement is unstoppable, and I am further convinced that the remarkable work undertaken by Professor Jacques Benvéniste, into the mechanisms of the action of homeopathic remedies, will have serious implications in the fields of biology and medicine.

It is the dream of every human being to pass from birth to death without any serious disease. In order to make this aspiration a reality, this book has been written with humility. Not everything is resolved and each of us has many more pages to write in the book of life.

1
The principles of homeopathy

I. Samuel Hahnemann (1755–1843)

The father of homeopathy

A disillusioned doctor

In 1779, at the age of 24, Samuel Hahnemann set up medical practice in Hettstadt, Saxony. He had been an outstanding student, and was able to translate Latin and Greek easily. In addition to his native German, he was fluent in French, Italian, and English.

However, he was a disillusioned doctor! Disappointed by his studies, he was rapidly disillusioned by the practice of medicine. A letter, written to his friends, illustrates the depth of his despair and bitterness: "Eight years of scrupulous care taken in medical practice had made me realize the futility of orthodox methods".

Six years of research

Human experimentation

In 1790, after 11 years of medical practice, which he believed to have been totally ineffectual, Samuel Hahnemann closed his surgery. He told his patients that he would forthwith devote his time and energy to experimentation and research.

However, in order to provide for his large family (he was to have 11 children in all), Hahnemann used his linguistic skills in translating a wide range of books. This is how he came to discover the works of the famous Albrecht von Haller, in particular his *Helvetian Pharmacopoeia*, in which he wrote:

Samuel Hahnemann began his medical practice with the methods described by Molière: bloodletting and purging.

Haunted by his ignorance and failures, Hahnemann closed his surgery, and supported his family by doing translations.

The principles of homeopathy

Hahnemann thought long and hard about human experimentation, a revolutionary concept for the times.

'The use of substances similar to the disease can restore health.'

"The unadulterated medicine must first be tried on a healthy subject. Once you have ascertained its smell and taste, give a small dose and observe all the effects produced: the pulse, temperature, breathing, and body secretions. On the basis of the symptoms produced in a healthy person, you can then progress to experiments on the sick."

Hahnemann thought long and hard about human experimentation, a revolutionary concept at the time. It was the translation of the work on cinchona, by the famous Scottish doctor William Cullen, which led to his brilliant discovery.

Cinchona
Cinchona had recently been introduced from South America and was currently in vogue as a medicine for the treatment of 'intermittent fevers'. (Quinine, a derivative of cinchona, is used today as a treatment and preventative for malaria.) There were a number of theories about its mode of action.

The first experiments
Hahnemann was unhappy about this form of treatment as he considered cinchona a poison, having previously taken it himself for a fever. During the translation, he discovered that Cullen attributed cinchona's action on intermittent fevers to 'its action as a stomach tonic'. Hahnemann was not satisfied with the explanation, finding it fanciful. Influenced by von Haller's theories, he decided to experiment on himself, taking the cinchona whilst he was healthy and free of fever. This experiment formed the basis of homeopathy.

The Law of Similars
At that time all doctors studied the works of the celebrated Hippocrates. Therefore Hahnemann was familiar with the famous Law of Similars, written in the fifth century BC. It states: "The use

Homeopathy encyclopedia

of substances similar to the disease can restore a sick person to a state of health." Since ancient times the similarity between a substance's toxicity and its healing power had been observed.

After confirming the effects of cinchona by experimenting on his friends, Hahnemann was positive that other substances could similarly yield results. He deduced that the study of the effects of a substance on a healthy individual would uncover its curative actions. He validated Hippocrates' Law of Similars with human experimentation.

The study of the effects of a substance on a healthy person allows for the discovery of its potential curative effects.

The founding text

Hahnemann's experiment with cinchona

"I took four drachmas [a contemporary unit of weight] of good cinchona, twice a day for several days. First I noticed coldness in my hands and feet. I became tired and sleepy. Then I developed palpitations; my pulse was strong and rapid. I experienced an intolerable anxiety and trembling, but without any chills. My limbs were weak, my head throbbed, my cheeks were red, and I was thirsty. In short, all the symptoms of an intermittent fever appeared one after another, but without any real fever. In my opinion, all the symptoms typical of intermittent fever appeared: the dulling of the senses, the stiffness of all the joints, but above all, the vague, unpleasant feeling within the bones. Each crisis lasted between two and three hours, and only recurred when I took another dose. I stopped taking the medicine and recovered my good health."

Hahnemann went on to note:

"Peruvian bark [cinchona] a remedy for intermittent fevers, works because it can produce symptoms similar to those of intermittent fever in healthy people.

"In order to cure certain types of intermittent fever, Peruvian bark must produce a type of artificial fever."

The principles of homeopathy

The experiments with cinchona could be repeated using other substances.

The birth of homeopathy, 1796

In 1796, Samuel Hahnemann published the results of six years of research in the most prestigious medical review of the day: Professor Hufeland's journal The article was entitled 'Essay on a new method for discovering the curative powers of medicinal substances, with observations on the principles apparent to date.'

An eventful life

From that time, Hahnemann resumed medical practice and rapidly achieved fame, but also became the object of jealousy and controversy. Alternately idolized and scorned, Hahnemann was criticized by some colleagues and supported by others. He had to move to another town several times. A tireless worker, he experimented unceasingly on new products and refined his therapeutic methods. He found countless cures and was emulated throughout Europe.

Hahnemann experimented unceasingly with new products and refined his therapeutic methods.

The Organon

From 1796 until his death in 1843, Hahnemann developed his doctrine, which he described in his most famous book, *The Organon*, which ran to six editions (the last one was published posthumously).

At the age of 73, Hahnemann published *Chronic Diseases*, a synthesis of his observations and reflections.

The triumphant final years in Paris

Widowed in 1830, he married a 30-year-old Frenchwoman in 1835. Melanie d'Hervilly had come from Germany to consult with him. He settled in Paris with her, practising for another eight years until his death. He was regarded as a great doctor by his healed patients, but was hated by the medical establishment whom he upset.

Homeopathy encyclopedia

Melanie and Samuel Hahnemann are buried in the Père-Lachaise cemetery in Paris, where devotees of homeopathy can make their posthumous tributes.

The glory of Hahnemann

Hahnemann is now world famous. Tens of thousands of doctors use his methods, developing and improving the techniques. However, his crowning achievement has still not been officially recognized: he was the first western doctor to break with the medical practices of the Middle Ages and initiate medical research.

2. The Law of Similars and infinitesimal doses

The founding principles

Source of the Law of Similars

As we have seen, Hippocrates, and not Hahnemann, postulated this law. He stated that: "The use of substances similar to the disease can restore health".

It proposes a parallel between the toxicological action of a substance and its therapeutic power. However, before Hahnemann, it had only been demonstrated in a minority of cases.

The eighteenth-century German doctor Georg Ernst Stahl wrote the following prophetic insight:

"I am convinced that diseases succumb to substances that cause a similar ailment. This is how I succeeded in treating the predisposition to heartburn with very small doses of sulphuric acid,

Hahnemann triumphed in Paris, adored by the people but detested by the members of the medical establishment.

Hahnemann's crowning achievement was to found medical research.

The principles of homeopathy

From material doses to infinitesimal doses: in order to minimize side effects, Hahnemann gradually progressed to the concept of diluting remedies.

when a variety of absorbent powders had been used in vain."

Hahnemann's application of the Law of Similars

This provided Hahnemann with the main theme of his work: human experimentation, and the relationship of his observations on the effects of known drugs with the Law of Similars. The latter demonstrated his genius.

He used the medicines current in his time, and observed that his subjects did not all react in the same way. It was necessary to vary the experimental conditions: the age and gender of the subjects, the dose of the medicine, etc.

He noted the symptoms, psychological and physical, subjective and objective, and also the 'modalities'. These are external or internal factors that can improve or aggravate the condition.

He studied the following groups of modalities, related to:

• Rhythm: time of day, season, and periodicity

• Environment: climate and atmospheric conditions

• Position: sitting, standing, lying down, doubled over

and their relationship with body functions: rest, sleep, movement, and the menstrual periods.

He also noted the aetiology – i.e. the infective and biological causes of disease, the psychological influences, climatic factors, the effects of nutrition, trauma, and toxicity.

Homeopathy encyclopedia

Thus he was able to define the 'pathogenesis', or causative factors, of each drug tested.

Infinitesimal doses

The Law of Similars does not specify the use of extremely diluted or infinitesimal doses. However, it is well known that homeopathic remedies contain a very small amount of the active substance. In high dilutions the active substance is non-existent, which leads one to assume that another process is responsible for its action, possibly electro-magnetic radiation.

When Hahnemann first used his remedies, he prescribed them in material doses. Over time, he discovered that he could prevent any unwanted side effects by diluting the remedies. Not only was the action maintained, it actually intensified with serial dilution.

Hahnemann invented this serial dilution of homeopathic remedies.

3. Pathogenesis and Materia Medica

The homeopathic bible

Pathogenesis

This is the name given in homeopathy for the complete study of a medicine.

It is composed of three parts:

• the observations made following accidental poisoning by a substance

The modalities are of prime importance in selecting an appropriate remedy.

Hahnemann invented the use of extreme dilutions of substances to avoid the toxic side effects of higher doses.

Each homeopathic remedy has a pathogenesis, which is the result of studying the effects of high doses on a human subject.

• the observations made following experimentation on healthy volunteers (provings)

• the clinical observations of homeopathic practitioners during the two hundred years of practice

All these symptoms are described in great detail, together with aggravating and ameliorating factors.

Each remedy has its own unique pathogenesis.

The homeopathic Materia Medica is a source of knowledge about the use of each remedy, for each person in a given situation.

Materia Medica

The books of homeopathic Materia Medica are collections of these pathogenetic profiles. There are a great number of them because in two hundred years countless authors have contributed their own observations and experimental work, based on the principles which were laid down by Hahnemann.

The most reputable and complete Materia Medica books are the constant companions of the homeopath, providing a source of information on numerous remedies and their applications in an individual or given situation.

There is also a wide range of simplified versions, which are more accessible to the general public. The third part of this book is one example of this type.

Homeopathy encyclopedia

4. The rules of homeopathy

The application of the Law of Similars

Homeopathy combines a therapeutic method with a different concept of the patient–doctor relationship. Both entail rules.

The therapeutic method

First rule

Every active substance that acts on the functions of the human body provokes a set of symptoms

---

An example of pathogenesis

The pathogenesis of ARNICA, an important remedy for trauma, is described in the Materia Medica written by Michel Guermonprez, Madeleine Pinkas, and Monique Torck:

• remedy with a general action

• the effect of trauma, strain, and overexertion: pain, bruising, haemorrhage, shock. Mechanical injury and the effects of stasis, traumatic pregnancies and deliveries, surgery

• Cardiovascular pathology: strain of the heart muscle, angina caused by exercise, high blood pressure, inflammation of the arteries with cramp brought on by exertion, painful varicose veins, fragile capillaries, strokes

• Exhaustion, depression, and despair brought on by physical, intellectual, and emotional challenges. Broken will, desire for solitude, paradoxical indifference

• Infectious and toxic states with a loss of energy and shock

• Febrile conditions: a dejected, prostrate, pessimistic patient, who does not react. Cardio-vascular failure

• Aggravating factors: trauma, overexertion and violent emotions. Worse for touch, speaking to the person, or even the presence of another person

• Ameliorating factors: lying face down, the application of hot compresses

The principles of homeopathy

The search for a suitable remedy follows a simple path: the comparison of the effects of a remedy on a healthy person, with the symptom pattern in a sick person. If the two patterns are similar or close, the remedy is used to treat the sick person.

The homeopathic doctor attaches great importance to establishing a highly personal relationship with the patient. Listening to a detailed description of the symptoms and the modalities requires consultations lasting 30 to 60 minutes

characteristic to that substance in a healthy, sensitive person.

For example, coffee causes an acceleration of the heart rate (tachycardia), increased urine output, and a nervous excitation, with insomnia and a heightening of the senses. These readily observed signs are known as symptoms.

Second rule
Every sick person exhibits a set of symptoms characteristic of his or her illness.

For example, a person exhausted by mental over-exertion presents with excitability, insomnia caused by flights of ideas, and increased sensitivity to noise, light, or light touch. There is often a tendency to tachycardia.

Conclusion
The cure, demonstrated by the disappearance of these symptoms, can be achieved by a prescription of a low or infinitesimal dose of a substance that would produce similar symptoms in a healthy person. Therefore, COFFEA 6C (dilute coffee) would assist or cure the above-mentioned patient.

The relationship with the patient
The knowledge of the detailed symptoms, together with the appropriate modalities, requires a profound ability to listen to the patient; this is an integral part of homeopathic practice.

The medical homeopath places great importance on the precise details of everyday ailments: the rhythm of the illness and ameliorating and aggravating factors. The homeopath will also spend a great deal of time in elucidating the full history and will try to comprehend the relationship between the different complaints the patient may have.

The physical examination is equally systematic, and includes looking for signs, particularly on the skin, which may assist in the selection of a remedy according to the Law of Similars.

5. The homeopathic consultation

A medicine for the individual

The unity of the individual

The process of the homeopathic consultation is truly revolutionary in the context of modern day medical practice. The individual is regarded in his or her entirety, which opposes the conventional medical model of multiple specialities, which fragment and divide the person. As a result of this fundamental belief, each homeopath must go back to the onset of illness with each patient and fully understand it; only in this way can an authentic healing relationship be established.

Each illness has meaning, and that meaning lies in the personal history of the individual. Far from being a machine whose parts can be changed, as a

Homeopathy is a form of medicine that treats the individual, in the fullest sense of the word. Each person is viewed in his or her entirety, and as a unique being.

Homeopathy is a therapeutic method that consists of giving a sick person a substance in low or infinitesimal doses, a substance which will provoke similar symptoms in a healthy individual.

Thus COFFEA, made by serial dilution of coffee, would be an appropriate remedy for the person whose symptoms were described in the second rule.

purely technical form of medicine would have us believe, a human being should always be considered within the entirety of the physical, physiological, cultural, and historic setting. This is what sets a homeopath apart, and this is why homeopathy is said to be holistic. To put it more simply and more fully, homeopathy is medicine for the individual.

The uniqueness of the individual

Science has now confirmed that each person is truly unique, except for identical (monozygotic) twins. With those exceptions each of us is biologically and psychologically unique. One of the paradoxes of modern medicine is that treatments are identical and standardized despite the differences in people, whereas homeopathy allows us to individualize the treatment. By researching the long list of available remedies, the precise remedy can be found that will be most suitable for the patient, given the history and symptoms.

6. The homeopathic remedy

Mineral, animal or plant but diluted

The Codex, which is the official book of the French Pharmacopoeia, defines a homeopathic remedy thus:

"The homeopathic remedy is a medicine obtained by successive dilutions, known as Hahnemannian dilutions."

So, as we can see, these products are not defined by the source material, but by a specific manufacturing process.

The homeopathic remedy

Homeopathy encyclopedia

Different sources

Contrary to a widely held belief, homeopathy is not 'plant medicine'.

Homeopathic remedies are made from sources from the three kingdoms of nature: animal, plant, and mineral, as can be seen in the examples in the box below.

For minerals, naturally occurring salts or chemicals are used, as well as mixtures of salts or complex preparations.

For plant remedies, alcoholic tinctures are prepared from the active part of the plant; these are known as mother tinctures.

For animal remedies, the whole animal can be used or its organs or secretions, diluted in alcohol.

Homeopathic remedies are made from source material of animal, plant or mineral origin.

Different origins

• The mineral kingdom
NATRUM MURIATICUM is prepared from common salt.
SULPHUR is prepared from the mineral sulphur.
CALCAREA CARBONICA is prepared from the impure middle third of the oyster shell
– In some countries the chemical is used.
PHOSPHORUS is prepared from red phosphorus
– Sometimes white phosphorous is used instead.
MERCURIUS SOLUBLIS/MERCURIUS VIVUS is made from soluble black oxide of mercury

• The plant kingdom
BELLADONNA is made from the whole plant Atropa belladonna, the deadly nightshade.
BRYONIA ALBA is made from the root of the white bryony.
THUJA OCCIDENTALIS is made from the fresh green twigs of the Thuja tree.
LYCOPODIUM is made from the dry spores of the club moss.

• The animal kingdom
APIS MELLIFICA is prepared from the whole bee.
LACHESIS MUTA is prepared from the venom of the South American bushmaster snake.
SEPIA is prepared from the ink of the cuttlefish.

The principles of homeopathy

The dilutions are made in a ratio of 1 part in 10 (X or D, decimal dilution) or 1 in 100 (C or centesimal scale). It takes considerable time to prepare a remedy from the mother tincture.

Most homeopathic remedies are made by this method.

The dilutions

It takes considerable time to prepare the remedies. There are two methods of preparation, starting with the mother tincture made from animal or plant origin.

Hahnemannian dilution

This method comprises serial dilution of 1 part of mother tincture in 9 or 99 parts of alcohol or water/alcohol mixture. It is the method used by Hahnemann himself, when he first started his practice, and strictly follows the procedure used in chemistry.

In practice, 1 millilitre of mother tincture is added to 99 millilitres of alcohol (or water/alcohol mixture) to make the first dilution of 1/100 (1C). One millilitre of this dilution is added to another 99 millilitres of alcohol, or water/alcohol mixture to make the 2C dilution. A clean flask is used for each dilution and the mixture is vigorously shaken, or succussed as it is known in homeopathy. This is done 30 times to obtain the 30C potency.

These dilutions are known as C potencies, C meaning centesimal. Belladonna 6C means that the remedy contains a solution that has been obtained from six serial dilutions and succussions from the mother tincture of the plant Atropa belladonna.

In the same way dilutions can be prepared with a dilution of 1 in 9 parts alcohol or water/alcohol mixture. These are known as D potencies (decimal) or X potencies.

M potencies have been diluted one part in 999 of alcohol or water/alcohol mixture.

Homeopathy encyclopedia

The Korsakov method

This method is commonly used in France. Using an automated machine, the mother tincture is progressively diluted in a single flask. The first dilution of 1 in 100 is placed in the flask. Then, and following each progressive dilution, the flask is vigorously shaken. It is automatically emptied and refilled with 100 drops of the solvent (water/alcohol mixture). The traces of each dilution that remain in the flask ensure the continuity of the process.

This process is obviously very imprecise. Little importance is placed on the dilution; rather the shaking or succussion is regarded to be important. It is essential to know the exact number of succussion cycles. LYCOPODIUM 10,000 K has been succussed 10,000 times.

The remedies prepared by this method certainly have different effects from those prepared by the Hahnemannian method. They have a more generalized effect.

The Korsakov method is not precise. However, it allows for thousands of dilutions and succussions. The remedies prepared in this way have a different effect from those prepared by the Hahnemannian method.

Triturations

Minerals, which are insoluble in water or alcohol are triturated; the material is made into fine powder by grinding it in lactose, using a pestle and mortar. The process is similar to that used in dilutions; 1 part of mineral is ground with 99 parts of lactose to obtain the first trituration. After the third serial trituration, the product is rendered soluble.

Triturations are reserved for minerals which are insoluble in water or alcohol.

Granules and tablets

Homeopathic remedies are usually sold in the form of tablets or granules coated with the active substance. They can be coated with different potencies of the remedy.

Granules or tablets of
lactose or sucrose are
coated with the different
dilutions to make the
remedies.

The homeopathic
remedy cannot be
altered in any way to
render it toxic.

Other products

Homeopathic remedies can be manufactured
from the mother tincture and serial dilutions into
a variety of pharmaceutical products: oral drops,
suppositories, injections, powders, pomades,
syrups.... In practice these are rarely used.

Expiry date

Homeopathic remedies, in the form of tablets or
granules, retain their potency for decades if
stored in a cool, dry environment away from
strong scents.

However, current legislation requires an expiry
date to be given for the products.

The homeopathic remedy cannot be altered in
any way to render it toxic.

The manufacture of remedies

Accredited homeopathic pharmacists may manu-
facture their own remedies, but many do not,
choosing to purchase from specialist manufacturers.
In France, the market is shared between two major
companies: Boiron and Pierre Fabre (who have
bought up Dolisos). They distribute their products
throughout France via numerous branches, and are
also active in many other countries.

Latin names

Homeopathic remedies are all given Latin names. This traditional practice has the
immense advantage of unifying all homeopathic prescriptions in the world.
Whether a homeopath is from France, England, Argentina, or India, the
prescription will be the same. This greatly enhances communication with foreign
colleagues, especially at international conferences.

These Latin names reflect the source of the remedy and are no more difficult to
remember than allopathic drug names, many of which were invented for
advertising purposes.

Remedies without prescribing instructions

Unlike conventional medicines, homeopathic remedies do not come with general prescribing information. The remedy is chosen on a highly individualized and meticulous study of the symptom picture. The information gathered from this detailed study must accurately reflect the homeopathic picture of the remedy, in accordance with the Law of Similars.

The information sheet for the remedy would therefore need to contain the entire Materia Medica of a remedy! This does not make it easy for the novice in homeopathy. Self-medication in homeopathy is much more difficult than in conventional medicine, where the products are labelled according to their precise properties, e.g. anti-spasmodic, analgesic, anti-inflammatory.

The control of the manufacturing process is as rigid as in any conventional pharmaceutical company.

7. Homeopathic complexes

Contradictory but useful

Homeopathic Complexes are mixtures of remedies (between 5 and 10 remedies), chosen for the similarities in their action. This may seem to contradict the laws of homeopathy, which demand the choice of an individualized remedy, specific to a particular situation. Therefore, it is hard to understand how these non-specific mixtures can work.

Homeopathic Complexes are mixtures of five to ten remedies, usually in low potencies, chosen for their synergistic action.

For the homeopathic novice

In fact, a qualified homeopath will never prescribe any homeopathic complexes. Indeed, he or she will always prescribe a remedy best suited to the individual, and it is a point of honour to prescribe as few remedies as possible. This is one of the criteria to be considered when selecting a good homeopath.

The principles of homeopathy

Homeopathic complexes are useful for self-medication in acute illnesses.

For acute conditions, take one tablet or granule every ten to fifteen minutes, until improvement occurs.

On the other hand, charlatans often prescribe complexes, as they appreciate the potential of homeopathy. It is far easier for the ignorant to obtain a result with a mixture of five to ten remedies, because there is a real possibility that the organism will differentiate between the various components and utilize the appropriate ingredients, whilst not reacting to those which are inappropriate.

Well made complexes

In fact, these complexes are well made, in that they combine within a tablet or granules, remedies that are closely related on a pathological basis. They are efficacious in acute illnesses, and are frequently used as a means of self-medication by patients who are unsure about selecting the correct remedy, preferring to take several with closely related indications.

This approach yields good results, because the organism seems to select the appropriate components. However, the remedies are in very low potencies, which makes them relatively ineffective in chronic long-standing complaints.

In brief

If you are starting to use homeopathy, use complexes for acute situations (colds, influenza, upper respiratory tract infections, attacks of nerves, travel sickness etc.)

If you are impressed by your first attempts at prescribing, learn to use each remedy from a popular guide, such as this.

In the case of a long-standing chronic complaint, consult a qualified medical homeopath, unless you have had extensive experience.

8. Rules governing dosage

How much, how often and what potency?

Acute or chronic illness: the dosage rules are different.

How many tablets?

The precise number of tablets is immaterial, as there is no direct relationship between the dose of a remedy and its effect. It is tempting to say that the quality is far more important than the quantity. However, it is customary to give recommendations regarding dosage. These can be changed without incurring any risk.

The difference between granules and tablets

There is no difference between the various homeopathic preparations – granules, tablets, or powders – in terms of their efficiency and action. It is a matter of personal preference.

How frequently and how often?

In acute conditions it is important to commence treatment as soon as possible after the first symptoms appear, and to continue treatment until there is an improvement. It is recommended that a tablet or granule be given every 15 minutes. When the condition is very acute, the remedy will often have to be repeated frequently.

In chronic conditions, low potency remedies are administered once or twice a day and higher potencies on a weekly or fortnightly basis. It is advisable to allow the remedies to dissolve in a clean mouth 15 minutes before breakfast and the evening meal.

The principles of homeopathy

Homeopathic remedies: catalysts to healing rather than medicines.

What potency?

The choice of potency is fundamental, and this causes problems for the novice. It is not always easy to obtain the different potencies outside specialist pharmacies.

It is necessary to consider the degree of similarity between the remedy and the individual. The higher potencies will have a greater effect on the whole person, including the emotional sphere.

Stopping treatment

In the case of acute conditions (upper respiratory tract infections, earaches, haemorrhoids) treatment should be stopped when the symptoms have disappeared.

In the case of long-standing chronic conditions, your homeopath will guide you with regard to the duration and frequency of treatment.

Contrary to common belief, treatment is not life long! Remedies act as catalysts to healing, as opposed to medicines in the conventional sense. This is why one can use them periodically to regain one's equilibrium and good health. A person whose health and liver function have been improved by LYCOPODIUM, for instance, can repeat it whenever their symptoms recur.

A case of tonsillitis

This morning, Juliet, aged 8, awakes complaining of a sore throat. She is not hungry, and feels lethargic. Her mother takes her temperature: 38.5 °C (101.3 °F). Using a torch and small spoon to depress the tongue, her mother notes that the throat is very red.

Juliet won't go to school today. She will have a tablet of BELLADONNA 6C and FERRUM PHOSPHORICUM 6C every 15 minutes. As soon as her mother notices an improvement, she will space out the remedies, giving them half-hourly, hourly and then every two hours.

Homeopathy encyclopedia

ARNICA – the great trauma remedy

- After a fall where a bruise develops: take ARNICA 6C

- After falling off a bicycle into a ditch and sustaining painful grazes and bruising to the arm and right leg: take ARNICA 30C

- After a car accident with multiple injuries, a broken wrist, a mild head injury, and emotional shock and fright: take ARNICA 30C repeatedly over a few days

---

Homeopathy seeks to restore the equilibrium and harmony of the individual.

9. Homeopathy and allopathy

Two opposing principles, which are compatible

Homeopathy and allopathy are based on opposing principles, but can be used to complement one another.

Most people are unaware that it was Hahnemann who coined the term 'allopathy' to distinguish the therapeutic method he had just invented from the medicine of his era. Ever since then, there has been a great deal of intolerance and bad feeling between the two opposing camps.

Compatibility between homeopathy and allopathy

Many patients ask whether they should discontinue their orthodox medication in order that the homeopathic remedies might act on a 'clean slate'. If this was the case, the medicine would have already had an effect, and no remedy would act following a previous allopathic intervention.

Homeopathic and allopathic remedies act very differently and do not have similar effects. In view of this fundamental difference, it is possible to use them in conjunction with one another, or at different times.

This concept runs contrary to all the findings of contemporary scientific knowledge, which has demonstrated that each active substance acts on a specific site. It is likely that this is also the case with homeopathic remedies, so it can be presumed that they will remain active even in the presence of another treatment.

In practice, it is often impossible to discontinue an orthodox treatment which was started months, if not years before. Notable examples would be the treatment of hypertension (high blood pressure), depression, epilepsy, and certain conditions requiring anti-coagulant therapy. All these conditions may be treated with homeopathy, and clinical experience has demonstrated that it can be sufficiently effective to allow a reduction, or in some cases gradual withdrawal, of allopathic treatment.

The opposite situation is also seen: a patient undergoing homeopathic treatment may require allopathic treatment for an acute condition. This can occur with children who are being treated for recurrent upper respiratory tract infections and bronchitis. One particular acute illness may require a short course of antibiotics, but this will not make it necessary to halt the homeopathic treatment.

The situation with cortisone and other steroids needs to be considered separately. It does seem that these drugs interfere with homeopathic treatment, making it less effective. It is therefore important to work with both types of treatment at the same time. It is possible to reduce the dramatic side effects of the steroids by using appropriate homeopathic remedies.

Homeopathy encyclopedia

Homeopathy and antibiotics

Homeopathic remedies do not have any antibacterial properties. This means they cannot directly destroy the bacteria in an infection. However, homeopathy claims to cure many infectious conditions. How can one explain this apparent paradox?

Infectious diseases are caused by bacteria, viruses, or parasites. Sore throats can be caused by an infection with Staphylococci bacteria, Staphylococci bacteria can cause boils and other infections. Infection with the poliomyelitis virus leads to the terrible paralyzing disease of polio. Herpes infection of the skin is due to the virus of the same name. Malaria is transmitted by parasites.

The aim of allopathic treatment is to kill the responsible organism. Antibiotics do precisely that, but they only kill bacteria. Other medicines are suitable for parasites, such as quinine for malaria. There are few drugs that can kill viruses. Acyclovir is effective for herpes, and there are certain anti-viral drugs that can be used in the treatment of AIDS, but none of them provides a cure.

Homeopathic remedies are not intended to kill the infective organism, as a consequence of their nature and dilution. They act by improving the person's natural defences against infection. This is an essential factor, entirely overlooked by conventional antibiotic therapy. It is not enough merely to kill off the infectious agent in order to resolve the condition. It could not have arisen in the first place unless there was an inherent susceptibility in the individual. This inherent susceptibility to infection is what concerns the homeopath.

Homeopaths therefore prescribe remedies in infections to help the individual fight back and destroy the infective agents, by using the body's natural defences. Thus the remedies are compatible with antibiotic treatment, as they act according to very different principles.

Side effects

Side effects are unwanted symptoms which occur during a course of treatment, and are unrelated to the desired therapeutic effect. They are frequently observed in classical allopathic treatment. For example, anti-inflammatory drugs used for rheumatic complaints frequently cause stomach pain.

Homeopathic remedies reactivate the individual's immune defences without having any undesirable side effects.

The reactivation of the immune defences can cause a slight resurgence or change in the symptoms after two or three weeks of homeopathic treatment.

Nosodes are deep acting remedies with a profound effect, especially on the immune system.

This does not happen with homeopathic treatment. The remedies do not have any undesirable side effects. This is a consequence of their very specific action (the Law of Similars) and the high dilutions employed.

However, patients may feel slightly worse after two or three weeks of treatment. This is not due to side effects, but to a reactivation of the immune defences, which can cause a temporary exacerbation of the symptoms. These symptoms are pre-existing, unlike in the case of allopathic medicines which throw up new and unrelated symptoms. These symptoms rapidly settle and a sense of well-being is restored.

10. Nosodes

Deep acting remedies which are highly individualized

Definition

Nosodes are more readily available in some countries than in others. In the UK, for example, there is no current legislation banning their use and they are always used in high potency.

Nosodes are prepared from infected material of plant or animal origin. As they are derived from secretions, excretions or tissues, they contain a mixture of components: some derived from the host, others from the infectious agent. They are named according to the source material.

Isopathic remedies are prepared from materials that cause an illness; e.g. potentized pollens are used for the treatment of hay fever.

Homeopathy encyclopedia

The nature of nosodes

As can be seen from the definition, these are clearly highly complex remedies.

They are very deep acting and are best left in the hands of the professional homeopath. They are generally used in relatively high potencies.

STAPHYLOCOCCINUM is obtained from a culture of the Staphylococcus bacteria, which cause a number of purulent infections, particularly of the skin.

PSORINUM is derived from scabies, a parasitic infection of the skin.

TUBERCULINUM BOVINUM is derived from a tubercular abscess of bovine origin.

INFLUENZINUM is prepared from a culture of the influenza virus.

Isopathic remedies

These are prepared from material that causes an illness. Homeopathic preparations of allergens are frequently used to treat allergy, and potentized remedies made from allopathic medicines can be used to treat the side effects of the medication.

The use of nosodes

These remedies, originally introduced by Hahnemann, do not strictly conform to the Law of Similars. Their use is based on the belief that these pathological substances, used in potency, will strengthen inherent weaknesses in a person and heal their propensity to certain diseases.

Some nosodes are used extensively by homeopaths. Some practitioners, working in isolated areas where few remedies are available, prescribe them almost exclusively, with very encouraging results.

However, they are not recommended in self-medication, as they can cause strong reactions.

Nosodes: not recommended for self-medication.

11. Homeopathy and acute diseases

Efficacious in an emergency

Homeopathic remedies in emergency situations

A true emergency always requires medical intervention. One must always call for a doctor in the case of a haemorrhage, loss of consciousness, convulsions, or a high fever. If surgery is not appropriate to the condition, medicines will be used.

In previous generations, homeopaths used remedies in emergency situations, often with considerable success. One must bear in mind that, in those days, there was little allopathic medicine could offer in the way of treatment.

Nowadays, allopathic medicine has a large number of drugs to alleviate conditions, albeit temporarily. It has an array of anti-inflammatory and anti-spasmodic drugs, analgesics, anti-coagulants etc. Thus it has gradually supplanted the role of homeopathy in emergencies, but this may not be entirely justified. Without denigrating the importance of these drugs, it is useful to reconsider the two types of approach to treatment. For example, people who have a violent reaction to wasp stings

Many pharmacies and health shops stock homeopathic remedies.

The homeopathic treatment of animals is powerful evidence for the efficacy of homeopathy.

Homeopathy is effective in acute disease and emergencies.

Some examples of the use of nosodes

• INFLUENZINUM can be used as a preventative for colds and influenza

• STAPHYLOCOCCINUM is useful to build up the defences of people prone to purulent infections, such as recurrent boils

• PSORINUM is often used by homeopaths when remedies have seemingly lost their curative power

Homeopathy encyclopedia

may develop immense swelling at the site of the sting. In certain cases, treatment with APIS MEL- LIFICA may have results comparable with that of steroid injections.

In all emergencies, whilst awaiting medical atten- tion, it is never inadvisable to give the appropri- ate homeopathic remedy. It will not interfere with any medication prescribed later.

The rapid action of homeopathic remedies

The main criticism of homeopathy, in both emer- gency situations and acute conditions is the assumption that it takes time to act. One of the comments frequently made in the consulting room is, "But, Doctor, homeopathy takes a long time to work!"

In fact, well-indicated remedies, given appropri- ately, can act very quickly, as rapidly as allopathic medicines, if not more so. In these situations, one has to give a tablet every 15 minutes until the symptoms abate. This is the way to treat the onset of flu, sore throats, ear infections, or upper respiratory tract infections.

APIS MELLIFICA: spectacular effects.

One tablet every 15 minutes until the symptoms abate.

Example: a nosebleed

Ten-year-old Sally wakes up in tears at 11p.m. She has a nosebleed, something that happens from time to time.

Her father applies gentle pressure to her nostrils, and gives her a tablet each of ARNICA 6C, MILLEFOLIUM 6C and CHINA 6C.

He repeats the remedies, as soon as the tablets dissolve.

Within an hour all is peaceful again. There will be no further problems for a while.

The treatment of chronic diseases best demonstrates the efficacy of constitutional homeopathic therapy.

12. Homeopathy and chronic diseases

The perfect field of use

The treatment of chronic diseases best demonstrates the efficacy of homeopathy. It is difficult to assess its effects as compared with allopathic treatment in this field. Homeopathy acts on a deeper level, affecting the constitution, and assists in the restoration of equilibrium of the normal body functions. Allopathy, on the other hand, alleviates the symptoms of disease, without an effect on the underlying causes. Allopathy can reduce the symptoms of an allergic attack or calm the pain caused by inflammation in a case of rheumatism. This is why symptoms can recur when allopathic treatment is stopped, and why there is no improvement in the general state of health.

Homeopathic treatment, on the other hand, aims to deal with the underlying causes of disease, thus preventing a return of the symptoms. One can thus understand why time is needed to achieve a stable condition.

It is unreasonable to expect a cure within a few days for a health complaint that has been present for years!

The more established the pathology, the longer treatment must be pursued. There are usually noticeable effects within the first three months of treatment, and the remedies are then administered less frequently as health returns.

13. Homeopathy and serious diseases

The results, the hopes and the impasses

Cancer and serious diseases

This is at the heart of the debate between allopathy and homeopathy. It can be obscured by unreasonable expectations from the general public. It must be stated that even skilful homeopathy will not cure advanced cancer, tuberculosis, kidney failure, or cirrhosis of the liver.

This clear position allows us to distance ourselves from certain practitioners who lead their patients to believe that homeopathy is a sort of panacea. Whether they result from a tragic misunderstanding or deliberate fraud, these notions cause considerable damage to homeopathy.

That is not to say that homeopathy has no role to play in the treatment of serious diseases. Quite the contrary! Clinical experience has demonstrated the usefulness of homeopathic remedies in alleviating the side effects of certain aggressive allopathic treatments, such as chemotherapy for cancer. It can also strengthen the body's immune system.

Homeopaths believe, although formal evidence is lacking at this time, that their remedies may contribute to the prevention of serious diseases, especially cancer, as the remedies aim to restore the body's state of equilibrium. The exciting challenge facing the homeopath is to assist each person to live without any serious disease, from the cradle to the grave, by means of modulating the body's natural defences. The homeopath's work

Homeopathic remedies do not produce any toxic effects or any side effects, unlike allopathic medicines. Long standing homeopathic treatment does not pose any dangers.

The principles of homeopathy

Many homeopaths believe that their treatment may prevent the development of serious diseases.

assists that of the conventional doctor, who will only get involved at a later stage once a diagnosis is made.

Bearing in mind the sensitivity of this matter, it should be pointed out, that the latest research in homeopathy (both theoretical and clinical) might hopefully lead to potential cures for certain serious diseases. The results still need validation, but are encouraging, especially in the field of immuno-therapy.

Genetic diseases: the impasse

Genetic diseases, like haemophilia (a serious disorder of blood clotting) are caused by a defect in the chromosomes. This disorder is passed onto future generations by the parents, and at the moment there is no medical treatment available to correct the abnormality in the chromosomes. It is, however, possible to treat the problems that are a consequence of the genetic anomaly.

The homeopath will be able to treat the symp-

An example: breast cancer

Isabel, aged 38, has just had an operation for cancer of the right breast. The cancer was removed in its entirety, but chemotherapy has been recommended as a preventative measure against recurrence. In order to support her through this treatment, which is detrimental to healthy and cancerous tissue alike, her homeopath prescribes a constitutional remedy:

• PULSATILLA 30C one tablet a week

• NUX VOMICA 6C and SULPHUR 6C to cleanse the body, one dose of each three times a day during chemotherapy, and once a day on other days

• SILICA 30C once a week to boost her immune system and assist with healing

Homeopathy encyclopedia

toms of a person with a genetic abnormality, just like any other person, but will not be able to cure or alter the underlying genetic abnormality in any way.

14. Practitioners and consumers

Who practises, who uses the remedies?

There is a growing interest in homeopathy and other forms of complementary medicine. The numbers of medically trained homeopaths are growing every year, as are the numbers of non-medically qualified practitioners.

The general public is becoming increasingly well informed about homeopathy. There are now numerous books and articles available, as well as 'word of mouth' reports extolling the results obtained with homeopathic remedies. Patients are more reluctant to submit themselves to certain treatments in allopathic medicine, and are looking for a more gentle, natural method of treatment. The huge increase in over-the-counter sales of homeopathic remedies (over 20 per cent per annum) reflects this trend.

Homeopathic practitioners

Homeopathy has existed for over 200 years, and there are different schools of thought as to its practice. There are three main groups.

The first group of homeopaths believe that only one remedy should be prescribed at a time, and that remedy should encapsulate the whole person. The prescription may change as the disease

Most remedies are enormously complex. A remedy made from a plant such as Belladonna or Bryonia contains hundreds of different chemicals. Even a remedy made from a mineral source like Calcarea phosphorica has a hugely complex composition due to the impurities in the salts. It may be that they are all complex prescribers after all, without even realizing it!

evolves, or circumstances change. These homeopaths are known as classical, constitutional, or Kentian prescribers. (The famous American homeopath, Dr. Kent, advocated this approach to treatment.) They follow Hahnemann's doctrine in its purest form. In Europe they are called 'unicists'.

The second group believes this position is theoretically perfect but that, in practice, it is very difficult to find a single remedy to cover all the patient's symptoms. Therefore they prescribe several medicines at a time, but confine themselves to as few as possible, usually between two and five. This approach is common in many European countries. They are known as 'pluralists' and also claim to follow the teachings of Hahnemann.

The third group believes that the body can differentiate from a mixture of remedies those components that are appropriate to the body's needs. Therefore, they prescribe mixtures of remedies, which cover a particular ailment rather than remedies specific to the patient. They are known as 'complex prescribers' and do not closely follow Hahnemann's teachings. Some of the homeopathic remedies on sale do, however, contain such complexes of remedies.

There are excellent homeopaths in all three schools of thought, and it is impossible to come down in favour of one approach rather than another within a few lines of text.

Practitioners and consumers

15. Homeopathy, trace elements, and vitamins

Very close and synergistic

Trace elements like copper, iron, magnesium, zinc, and manganese, and vitamins such as vitamin A, E, C, and B1, are found in very small quantities in the body, yet they are essential to life. They are known collectively as 'micro-nutrients'.

They ensure the smooth function of the thousands of chemical reactions that are occurring continually in the human body. They act as catalysts, which means they facilitate the chemical reaction without being used up or destroyed in the process.

The body requires only minute amounts of these micro-nutrients; they must be present in a usable form to ensure the normal function of the body.

Many of these micro-nutrients are used in homeopathic potencies. For example, copper is prescribed under the name Cuprum metallicum, and is useful for the treatment of cramp. Manganese is prescribed as Manganum, cobalt as Cobaltum and zinc as Zincum.

Vitamins are not available in homeopathic potencies. When prescribed in material doses, they may assist in restoring metabolic equilibrium in certain diseases.

Many homeopaths prescribe micro-nutrients as an adjunct to their treatment.

Trace elements and vitamins are essential in small quantities for maintaining the thousands of chemical reactions that occur within our cells. They act as catalysts to these processes.

Micro-nutrients help to maintain good health.

The micro-nutrients

These are classified into two groups:

• Trace elements: Aluminium, Antimony, Arsenic, Boron, Chromium, Copper, Fluoride, Iodine, Iron, Lithium, Magnesium, Manganese, Molybdenum, Nickel, Selenium, Silica, Tin, Vanadium, and Zinc

• Fat soluble vitamins: vitamin A (Retinol), vitamin B12, vitamin D (Calciferol), vitamin E (Tocopherol), and vitamin K

• Water soluble vitamins: vitamin B1 (Thiamine), vitamin B2 (Riboflavine), Niacin, Pantothenic acid, vitamin B6 (Pyridoxine), Biotin, Folic acid, vitamin C (Ascorbic acid) and b-carotenes

---

Acupuncture is an ancient traditional form of medicine.

16. Homeopathy and acupuncture

Perfectly compatible

Many homeopaths also use acupuncture in their treatment. This is justified once there is an understanding of the nature of this ancient Chinese medicine. Acupuncture is not administered in isolation in the Far East. On the contrary, it is one of the components of traditional Chinese medicine, which is divided into five levels of treatment:

Level 1 Use of energy, known as Chi energy

Level 2 Use of diet and hygiene

Level 3 Use of medicines

Level 4 Use of acupuncture and moxibustion

Level 5 Use of surgery

According to eastern philosophy, the quality of these treatments decreases from level 1 to 5. The

Homeopathy encyclopedia

use of medicines lies at level 3. They are intended to have a profound effect on the regulation of the life energy. Homeopathic remedies fit into this level of treatment as they have an equally profound effect on the body.

17. Homeopathy and vaccination

A source of potential conflict

Ever since Edward Jenner first discovered the smallpox vaccine in 1798, the use of vaccination to prevent epidemics and to enhance the body's resistance to disease has met with mixed success. Vaccines are not all equally effective, and there is constant research to improve them.

The issue of vaccination provokes strong opinions within the medical profession and in the general public, regarding its efficiency, appropriateness, and safety.

The homeopathic viewpoint

Contrary to common belief, there is no such thing as a homeopathic vaccine. There are certain remedies that can be used to enhance the body's defences against the cold and flu viruses, such as Anti Cold and Flu remedy and Influenzinum. These do not produce antibodies, unlike the classical vaccinations.

Where vaccination is compulsory, such as yellow fever when travelling to South America, there is no contra-indication during on-going homeopathic treatment. Remedies may be prescribed to counteract some of the more unpleasant effects of vaccination.

Vaccines vary in their efficiency and safety profile.

There are no homeopathic vaccines.

18. Special precautions

False perceptions

Misconceptions abound about homeopathy, and, although there may be a grain of truth in some of the stories, they are often distorted and exaggerated out of all proportion.

Tablets under the tongue?

This recommendation stems from the desire to allow the active ingredients in the remedy to pass directly into the bloodstream, thus bypassing the digestive tract and liver. The stomach contains a highly acidic liquid, which may adversely affect some medications. The liver acts to detoxify the body.

Absorption under the tongue is therefore the best way to protect the medicine. However, homeopathic remedies are still effective when swallowed. In young children, remedies dissolved in their feeding bottle still give excellent results.

In veterinary medicine, the remedy is generally mixed into the food without any appreciable alteration in its effects. This is very fortunate. It would be hard to imagine vets trying to force a tablet into the mouth of every chicken on a farm!

Mint

This is a frequently questioned substance. Since the start of homeopathy, mint has been forbidden during homeopathic treatment. This prohibition was started by Hahnemann himself, who mentioned it in his book The Chronic Diseases in 1832, in the middle of a long list of prohibited substances: perfumes, scented water, aromatic infusions, aniseed, throat lozenges, liqueurs, chocolates,

---

Remedies to counteract the side effects of vaccines? Thuja may be helpful – see Thuja in Section 3

The best way to absorb the remedy is to place it under the tongue to dissolve. However, it is still effective if swallowed.

Mint does not always have the detrimental effect on remedies that is often believed.

Homeopathy encyclopedia

dental powders, and tinctures. Curiously, there is no mention of mint in the sixth and final edition of *The Organon*. There is, however, a long list of prohibited substances and practices: "the wearing of woollen garments against the skin, a sedentary lifestyle in foul air, excessive breast feeding, nightlife, lack of personal hygiene, unnatural pleasures, excitation from erotic books, masturbation, and coitus interruptus".

It is difficult to see why mint has captured the public imagination to such an extent that it has maintained its status as a banned substance. Hahnemann's strictures were logical in his time: from the advice on diet and personal hygiene on the one hand, to the avoidance of products that were believed to have a therapeutic effect on the other.

We now know that mint does have beneficial effects. Experiments performed on guinea pigs, by Professor Bastide at the Faculty of Pharmacy in Montpelier, seem to show that there is no adverse effect on homeopathic remedies following the use of mint... at least in animals!

In short, this prohibition should be taken lightly. Our patients should not be terrified to take peppermint tea during their treatment, as clinical experience shows this not to be detrimental to their remedies.

Do not touch the remedies with your hands

This is another common belief. Perhaps it is because it touches on the important matter of the nature of the homeopathic remedies. Are the remedies delicate as they contain an immeasurable amount of the active substance? Are they not really matter at all? If that were indeed so,

Homeopathic remedies can be touched without a detrimental effect on their activity.

Homeopathic treatment is free from the risks of toxicity (even after excessive consumption) and serious side effects.

could handling them alter their structure in some way and hence their efficacy?

It is important to be clear about this. The remedies are a material reality, even if science cannot yet determine their precise nature. The structure of the tablets is such that they are impregnated with the active remedy, right to their core. They can be handled without risk.

19. The risks of homeopathy

No risks, no side effects

Accidental ingestion

"Doctor, My son has just swallowed a bottle of Belladonna 6C. What should I do?"

There is nothing to do. Just keep calm, and avoid calling the nearest poisons unit! Homeopathic remedies are never toxic, because of their extreme dilution.

There are two potential scenarios:

One: The child has no ill effects at all. He's perfectly well and has swallowed the tablets of Belladonna by accident. In view of his good health, the Belladonna will have no effect on him, and nothing untoward will happen.

Two: The child is being treated with Belladonna for a sore throat. The only consequence of taking a large amount of the remedy is a possible intensification of his symptoms. This will be short-lived and is not dangerous in any way. It will pass very quickly.

Homeopathy encyclopedia

Contra-indications

As we have seen, homeopathic remedies are never toxic in potency.

However, some remedies should be treated with care. They act by stimulating the body's defence system, and if the stimulus is too strong for the individual this may lead to an inappropriate, or even counter-productive, effect.

A typical example is the use of Hepar sulph in low potency. This remedy assists in pus formation, which may be inappropriate if pus is forming in a closed body cavity.

There are no formal contra-indications to the use of homeopathy. It is, however, essential to use the correct potencies of the correct remedies. This may be difficult in cases of self-medication.

If you have any doubt about the diagnosis, or the appropriateness of self-medication, please contact your doctor or homeopathic physician. This book is designed to help you treat minor ailments and professional advice should always be sought if you are in doubt.

There are no contra-indications to homeopathic treatment.

The less toxic the individual's system is, the more effective homeopathy will be.

20. Homeopathy and toxic substances

The influence of toxins

Tea, coffee, and tobacco

Tea, coffee, and tobacco are toxic substances whose effects vary from individual to individual. As homeopathy aims to regulate, harmonize, and detoxify the body, it is logical to consider whether

Build up a homeopathic first aid pack. It is not expensive and can be used to treat a variety of conditions when they start. The remedies are effective for years and can be replaced when they run out. There are sufficient granules or tablets in each tube for several uses.

these substances may interfere with the action of the remedies.

Homeopaths have noticed that homeopathy does not work as well when there is toxicity present. The explanation for this observation does not lie in the reaction of the remedy with the toxin, but more in the profound imbalance caused by the toxin. This is what makes it difficult for the remedy to act properly.

Maybe this is why homeopathy is so effective in young children. They have been less exposed to toxins, and one could say they are less 'messed up'.

Patients are advised not to smoke or drink coffee for an hour prior to taking a remedy and for an hour afterwards. These toxic substances may potentially interfere with the absorption of the remedy from the mouth.

21. The first aid kit

Get one as soon as possible

In homeopathy, self-medication is only possible if you have the remedies to hand. It cannot be stressed enough that the remedies should be taken immediately at the start of an illness. This is only practical if one has a little homeopathic kit to hand. Illnesses always seem to strike when the pharmacies are closed, the doctor's answerphone is on, or you're stranded in the countryside, miles from civilization!

This section is designed to help you put together one or two first aid kits, so that you can deal with any little emergencies as they arise. You can use these remedies, given the indications in this book, whilst awaiting a consultation with your homeopath.

Homeopathy encyclopedia

The basic kit

This consists of 20 remedies:

ACONITUM NAPELLUS 6C: the onset of colds, coughs, fevers, upper respiratory tract infections, sinusitis, palpitations, and overexertion.

APIS MELLIFICA 6C: burns, conjunctivitis, chilblains, herpes, insect stings, shingles, sunburn, mild sunstroke, sore throats, tonsillitis, swollen joints, and hives.

ARNICA MONTANA 6C: aches, cramps, the after-effects of trauma, dental work and surgery, burns, haemorrhoids (piles), laryngitis, inflammations of joints and tendons, and over-exertion.

ARSENICUM ALBUM 6C: diarrhoea, ear infections, indigestion, and shingles.

BELLADONNA 6C: abscesses, burns, conjunctivitis, ear infections, impacted earwax, fevers, German measles, measles, mumps, scarlet fever, and sunstroke.

CALENDULA 6C: abscesses, acne, burns, chilblains, eczema, nappy rash, impacted earwax, insect bites, and wounds.

CHINA OFFICINALIS 6C: abdominal bloating with digestive problems, diarrhoea, minor haemorrhages, and nosebleeds.

COLOCYNTHIS 6C: colitis, cramps, spasms, irritability, and period problems.

EUPATORIUM PERFOLIATUM 6C: influenza.

FERRUM PHOSPHORICUM 6C: abscesses, ear infections, feverish states, German measles, measles, sore throats and tonsillitis, and styes.

HYPERICUM 6C: sciatica, neuralgia, toothaches, and wounds.

IGNATIA AMARA 6C: abdominal bloating due to digestive problems, emotional and nervous states, irritability, gallstones, and overwork.

MERCURIUS VIVUS 6C: chickenpox, fevers, sore throats and tonsillitis, and mumps.

MILLEFOLIUM 6C: nosebleeds.

MOSCHUS 6C: nervous states, palpitations, and dizziness.

OSCILLOCOCCINUM 30C: the onset of flu.

PULSATILLA 6C: upper respiratory tract infections, pins and needles in the hands and feet, intolerance to fatty foods, mumps, and styes.

STAPHSAGRIA 6C: irritability, styes and wounds.

SYMPHYTUM 6C: to assist fracture healing.

TABACUM (or COCCULUS) 6C: travel-sickness.

Guide to the different methods

Back-up kit

There are a further 15 remedies in this pack, making a total of 35 remedies:

ALLIUM CEPA 6C: colds, upper respiratory tract infections, and sinusitis.

ANTIMONIUM CRUDUM 6C: diarrhoea, indigestion, varicose veins, and verruccas.

AMBRA GRISEA 6C: emotional and nervous states, palpitations.

BRYONIA ALBA 6C: asthma, cough, indigestion, flu, measles, and swollen joints.

CHAMOMILLA 6C: irritability, toothache, period problems and overexertion.

CUPRUM METALLICUM 6C: asthma, cough, cramps, stomach cramps, and over-exertion.

GELSEMIUM SEMPERVIRENS 6C: dizziness, emotional states, stage fright, eyestrain, flu, palpitations, and overexertion.

LEDUM PALUSTRE 6C: insect bites or stings, and puncture wounds.

LYCOPODIUM 6C: disorders of the liver and gall bladder.

NUX VOMICA 6C: constipation, dizziness, overindulgence in food and alcohol, haemorrhoids, indigestion, sleep problems, stiffness, and overwork.

OPIUM 6C: constipation.

RHUS TOXICODENDRON 6C: aching, stiff joints, trauma to the joints and tendons, stiff neck, flu, laryngitis, chickenpox, herpes, and shingles.

RUTA GRAVEOLENS 6C: trauma to the joints.

STRAMONIUM 6C: anger, excitability and worm infections (threadworm)

VERATRUM ALBUM 6C: diarrhoea, indigestion, travel-sickness, and period problems.

22. Belief in homeopathy

Homeopathy and the placebo effect

Homeopathy only works if you believe in it – doesn't it? This rather pointed question implies that homeopathy is nothing more than the placebo effect.

What is the placebo effect? Neutral substances are known to bring about a therapeutic effect in some individuals, despite the fact they do not contain any active ingredients. This is well recognized in allopathic medicine. Drug companies design tablets to take advantage of this unexplained effect. Responses to medication vary with the colour and size of the tablet used.

It is therefore reasonable to assume that there is a placebo effect in homeopathy, in common with all other types of treatment. This should not prejudice one's opinion of homeopathy. In this respect, homeopathic remedies do not differ from any other type of medication.

The placebo effect is poorly understood and is thought to be psychological. So why is it believed that this is the only effect of homeopathy? It is assumed that, because of the extreme dilution of remedies, there cannot be any active substance contained within them.

However, there are two situations where the placebo effect can be almost disregarded: the treatment of babies and animals. One can clearly demonstrate the efficacy of homeopathy in these two groups. It is difficult to imagine the placebo effect acting in cows or chickens!

The placebo effect is no more of an issue in homeopathy than it is in allopathy.

Merely believing that a remedy will heal you is not enough; to bring about a cure, the correct remedy must be taken appropriately.

World wide, Europe has the most followers of homeopathy.

Homeopathy is recognized in many countries. In the United Kingdom. the late Queen Mother was a firm believer and was regularly treated by her homeopath.

23. Homeopathy world wide

A growing practice

Europe

Homeopathy is practised in many European countries and is growing rapidly. There have been two European directives officially recognizing homeopathic medicine (in 1993 and 1995), and money has been allocated to research into the field.

In Germany, the term 'homeopathic doctor' is recognized by the medical association. Over 1,000 doctors hold this qualification, and there are a further 2,500 health care professionals licensed to prescribe homeopathy, known as 'heilpratiker'.

Homeopathy is not formally recognized in Belgium, but there are at least 150 doctors using it in their daily practice.

Homeopathy was introduced into the Netherlands over 150 years ago, and several hundred doctors practise it. Although highly regarded by the general public, it still lacks official recognition. Medical students are allowed to choose homeopathy as the subject of their thesis.

In Austria, homeopathy is recognized by the Ministry of Health. Some 300 doctors regularly prescribe homeopathy.

Homeopathy almost disappeared in Spain for a time, but there has been renewed interest in it since 1980. Many books on homeopathy have been translated and published in Spanish, demonstrating an appeal to the general public. There are about 200 practising homeopaths in Spain, some of them of French origin.

Homeopathy encyclopedia

In the United Kingdom, homeopathy is available within the National Heath Service, and the Faculty of Homeopathy was recognized in 1950 by an Act of Parliament.

In Greece, homeopathy was virtually unknown until its introduction in 1965 by a non-medical homeopath, who set up a private training school in Athens. About 50 doctors practise homeopathy, which is tolerated by the medical establishment.

In Italy, homeopathy is not recognized by the medical authorities or the insurance companies. Despite this, 400 doctors work as homeopaths.

Homeopathy was introduced to Sweden in 1826, but it still lacks formal recognition. An association was set up to promote homeopathy in Scandinavia (Sweden, Norway and Denmark). Of its 150 members, a hundred practitioners come from Sweden.

The history and development of homeopathy in Switzerland is linked to that of France. Only doctors may practice homeopathy, and insurance companies do not reimburse the cost of the remedies. Training schools are private, and there is close collaboration with the French. Approximately 50 doctors are trained homeopaths.

Although homeopathy is recognized in Russia, it is not practised much. There are about 500 homeopathic doctors, but this number has been growing annually since the fall of communism in 1989. There has been a veritable renaissance in other former Eastern block countries, such as Hungary, Poland, Romania, the Czech Republic, and Slovakia. Specialist laboratories have been set up and doctors are calling for formal training.

Homeopathy has developed in Russia following the collapse of Communism.

Homeopathy is becoming more popular in the United States of America.

A world first: homeopathy is part of the medical curriculum in Brazil.

The Americas

In the United States of America there was a golden age for homeopathy in the 19th and early 20th centuries. In 1930 there were 10,000 practising homeopathic doctors, and 9,000,000 people took remedies. There were two training colleges and 48 homeopathic hospitals and clinics.

Between 1930 and 1960 there were huge scientific advances in allopathic medicine. Homeopaths were fighting amongst themselves about the fundamental principles of homeopathy, and also fighting the medical establishment. These factors all served to sway public opinion away from homeopathy.

Since 1960, there has been a renewed interest in homeopathy, perhaps as a backlash to the increasingly technological and scientific approach of allopathic medicine.

Homeopathy is recognized in some states of America, and over 500 doctors practise it. Companies manufacturing homeopathic remedies have been set up.

Since 1895, homeopathic training and practice have been recognized in Mexico. There are over 500 medical practitioners and a national homeopathic hospital.

Homeopathy was introduced to Argentina only relatively recently, in 1930. Official recognition is still lacking, but there are over 500 homeopathic physicians, with another 2,500 doctors occasionally using the remedies. According to the federation of homeopathic laboratories in Argentina, a large proportion of the public use homeopathy.

Homeopathy encyclopedia

The introduction of homeopathy to Brazil dates back to 1818. On 25 September 1918, it was officially recognized by decree. It was declared a medical speciality on 28 July 1979. There are 200 homeopathic doctors, and the discipline is taught in the government medical school in Rio de Janeiro. There are four chairs of homeopathy. Since August 1999, the study of homeopathy has become a compulsory part of medical training.

The Ministry of Health in Chile has authorized homeopathic practice and treatment. There are about 30 doctors regularly using it.

Asia

In India, homeopathy is accepted on a par with allopathy and their traditional medicine (Ayruvedic medicine.) There are about 100 qualified homeopathic physicians there, as well as a very large number of practitioners who do not hold recognized medical degrees. Many of them have studied a medical course combined with homeopathic studies, but this training is not recognized outside the country.

In countries of the Far East (China, Japan, Korea, Indonesia, the Philippines, etc.) homeopathy is virtually unknown. This situation is set to change.

• The Faculty of homeopathy has just set up training in Japan

Africa

Homeopathy has had little impact in Africa, with the possible exception of Nigeria, Ghana, and South Africa. Many practitioners there are not medically qualified.

Homeopathy is virtually unknown in the Far East and most of Africa.

The work of Professor Jacques Benveniste demonstrates that biological information can be conveyed by electro-magnetic means. This may be a possible explanation of the mechanism of action of homeopathy.

Australasia

Since 1975, qualified doctors have been licensed to practice homeopathy, and a few dozen use it regularly.

There is no current legislation in New Zealand regarding homeopathy, but the government is not hostile to it. Interest has been growing since 1978, but the exact numbers of practitioners are unknown.

24. Research: what progress is being made?

A good question in the 21st century

Very little is known about the precise mechanism of action of homeopathy. The difficulty lies in the minute quantities used, and the problem of tracing them in the human body. For a long time we have had to be satisfied with hypotheses. Dr. Michel Durand summed up the situation, in the thesis he submitted in 1978:

"The action of a homeopathic remedy does not seem to be related to the amount of the substance contained within it. There is an immediate effect, which seems to be of an energetic nature.

There are two hypotheses proposed:

1) Molecules of the original matter are still present, but the preparation process somehow alters their chemical or physical structure.

2) There are no molecules remaining from the original material. The solvent is modified in some way to carry energetic information."

Homeopathy encyclopedia

Twenty years have passed since this was written, and it seems the second hypothesis is the more likely. The exciting and convincing work of Professor Jacques Benvéniste has demonstrated that homeopathic remedies do have a biological action *in vitro* under laboratory conditions.

Other independent researchers have recently validated his findings. As yet we do not know how this occurs. Biological fluids are mainly composed of water, and the explanation may lie in an alteration in the structure of the water molecules. Benvéniste coined the phrase 'the memory of water' to explain this phenomenon. He found himself a target for intense criticism within the scientific community, who were opposed to his radical ideas.

The concept that biological information may be transmitted by electro-magnetic means was regarded as revolutionary, despite the fact that all scientific break-throughs have been denounced initially as revolutionary. This work opens up a new field for research; a field that could be called 'electro-magnetic micro-pharmacology'.

Clinical research

Fortunately, homeopathy can fall back on clinical research, which has been continuing for over 30 years. Countless double-blind trials have demonstrated the efficacy of homeopathic remedies against allopathic medicines. The prestigious medical journal, *The Lancet*, published the results of an analysis of 89 homeopathic studies. The authors concluded that the results were "not compatible with the hypothesis that the clinical results of homeopathy are completely due to placebo".

Many studies have demonstrated the efficacy of homeopathic remedies against allopathic medicines.

2
Looking after yourself

Warning

This section contains advice on self-medication. The symptoms and diseases are listed in alphabetical order. To simplify matters, it is suggested that one tablet is used as a dose, which can be repeated as necessary according to results obtained.

Homeopathic remedies should only be used where the diagnosis is clear. If there is any doubt as to the nature of the illness, or it is serious, seek medical advice immediately.

Abdominal bloating

See 'Digestive disorders'.

Abdominal pain

See 'Digestive disorders'.

Abscesses and boils

A hard, red, painful swelling, often with a white head, is caused by accumulations of pus under the skin. Bacterial infection is present.

Add 10 drops of CALENDULA mother tincture to a cup of cooled boiled water and, using clean cotton wool, apply compresses to the infected area several times a day.

As soon as the first symptoms appear, take one tablet of each of the following remedies: BELLADONNA 6C, FERRUM PHOSPHORICUM 6C, and APIS 6C hourly. As soon as there is an improvement, reduce the frequency of taking the remedies.

If the abscess has already formed, take HEPAR SULPH 6C, one tablet three times a day to encourage the release of pus.

Homeopathy is compatible with antibiotic therapy, if it is recommended.

Warning

An abscess that takes a long time to heal, or multiple boils appearing within a short space of time, may be indicative of an underlying health problem. Seek medical advice if this occurs.

Abscesses on the face are potentially dangerous, and require immediate medical attention.

Absent periods (Amenorrhoea)

See 'Period problems'.

Accidents

See 'Trauma and burns'.

Aching muscles

Generalized muscular aching after unaccustomed exercise can be treated with ARNICA 6C and RHUS TOXICO-DENDRON 6C, one tablet three times a day. See 'Fever'.

Acne

See under 'Puberty and juvenile acne'.

Acute rheumatic fever

This condition has fortunately become rare since antibiotics were introduced. It is caused by an infection with the Streptococcus bacterium, and is characterized by swollen joints, rashes, and inflammation of the heart. It must be treated by a doctor, who will prescribe antibiotics and anti-inflammatory drugs.

Agoraphobia

This fear of open spaces and public places responds well to ARGENTUM NITRICUM 6C, used morning and evening, and before going out. Constitutional treatment may be helpful. Alternate ARGENTUM NITRICUM 30C and ACONITE 30C on a weekly basis.

Alcohol abuse

An occasional binge of alcohol may cause problems from the associated behaviour (fights, car accidents etc.). This may be more serious than the effects of the alcohol itself.

NUX VOMICA 6C, AGARICUS MUSCARIUS 6C, and STRAMONIUM 6C, one tablet of each taken every 15 minutes can reduce the feeling of inebriation.

Warning
Please note that the blood alcohol level will not be reduced although you may feel less drunk. Never drive after alcohol.

Chronic alcoholism: this is a serious disease requiring medical and psychological treatment. One should consult a homeopath for advice on a constitutional approach to the problem.

In the meantime three remedies may offer some assistance: NUX VOMICA 30C, one dose a week, SULPHURIC ACID 6C each night, and LACHESIS 6C each morning.

Allergies

Allergies are caused by an abnormal sensitivity to a substance known as an 'allergen'. Allergens can be inhaled (dust, pollen, feathers, or animal fur), ingested (foods, food additives, or medicines), come into direct contact with the skin (detergents, cosmetics, or household cleaning products) or may be injected (insect bites, injections, infusions, or vaccines.). This can lead to well known allergic states: asthma, contact dermatitis and certain types of eczema, urticaria, allergic rhinitis, and hay fever. Constitutional treatment by a homeopath is required to clear the tendency to allergies.

Avoid known allergens as much as possible.

HISTAMINE 6C every quarter of an hour may be useful along with the potentized allergen if known, e.g. mixed pollens and grasses, animal fur etc.

Alopecia (hair loss)

See 'Skin, hair, and nails'.

Altitude sickness (mountain sickness)

Certain people who are sensitive to the low oxygen composition of air at high altitudes will experience ringing in the ears, vertigo, headaches, breathlessness, fatigue, palpitations, insomnia, and anxiety.

These symptoms often settle once you acclimatize to the air. Take plenty of rest, avoid excessive activity, and eat light meals.

COCA 6C three times a day can speed up the acclimatization process.

For fear of heights, take GELSEMIUM 6C in the morning and evening, starting on the day before the trip.

Warning

If the symptoms do not settle quickly or there is an underlying chest or heart problem, seek medical advice from the nearest medical centre as soon as possible.

Anaemia

Anaemia is characterized by a reduction of red blood cells and haemoglobin (the molecule that carries the oxygen). Medical investigations are necessary to discover the cause of the anaemia.

If there was any known blood loss in the preceding weeks, CHINA 6C and FERRUM METALLICUM 6C one tablet, morning and night may be taken whilst awaiting treatment, after investigations.

Anal Fissures

See 'Haemorrhages and bleeding'.

Anal itching or inflammation (pruritus ani)

Anal itching (pruritus): this is often resistant to treatment. Try TEUCRIUM MARUM 6C twice daily, morning and evening, for several weeks.

Inflammation of the anal region: AES-CULUS 6C, ARNICA 6C, HAMAMELIS 6C and HURA BRASILENSIS 6C, one tablet of each four times a day.

See also anal fissures in 'Haemorrhages and bleeding'.

Angina pectoris

Spasm or obstruction of the coronary vessels, which carry oxygen to the heart muscle, lead to crushing chest pain. This is a medical emergency and a doctor or ambulance must be called immediately.

In a diagnosed case, where medical treatment has been started and all investigations have been performed, one could try ARNICA 6C and CACTUS GRANDIFLORUS 6C every 15 minutes.

Animal bites

See 'Trauma and burns'.

Anorexia nervosa

Anorexia nervosa is a reduction or total loss of appetite. It is a psychological condition. Weight loss may be severe, leading to malnutrition, and the immune system is compromised as a result.

A doctor must be consulted to exclude any physical causes for the loss of appetite and to assist with the treatment of the psychological state. Home-opathy may be useful in assisting other forms of treatment.

- In infants: LYCOPODIUM 6C, one tablet three times a week

- Anorexia with a tendency to withdrawal and isolation: NATRUM MURIATICUM 30C twice a week

- Anorexia with depression: SEPIA 30C twice a week

- Anorexia with changeable moods in girls who need a lot of comfort: PULSATILLA 30C twice a week

- Anorexia alternating with bulimia: ANTIMONIUM CRUDUM 30C and NUX VOMICA 30C twice a week

Warning
This condition requires expert medical advice and psychological support.

Anti-depressants

These drugs do cause problems with dependency and are prescribed in very high numbers in the western world. Their use is justified in some serious cases of depression.

A homeopath may assist with the treatment of the depression and assist with the reduction, or in some cases, withdrawal of these drugs.

Anxiety

See 'Nerves, fear, and anxiety'.

Arteriosclerosis (hardening of the arteries)

The blood vessels may become thickened and hardened due to a variety of factors. Fat is deposited within the vessel wall, leading to a reduction of blood flow to essential organs (heart, brain, etc.)

Following the diagnosis, regular treatment from a homeopath will be needed.
• As a preventative measure one can use PULSATILLA 6C, ARNICA 6C, and SECALE CORNUTUM 6C twice a week

When there is reduction of blood flow to legs, painful cramps may develop whilst walking. Medical advice should be sought as soon as possible. If you smoke, give up immediately. SECALE CORNUTUM 6C and NUX VOMICA 6C may help with the cramps.

The Mediterranean diet is recommended: fresh fish, lots of fruit and vegetables, cereals and whole grains should be eaten. A small amount of wine is thought to be beneficial. Red meat, dairy products, refined sugars and processed foods should be avoided.

Arthritis – inflammatory

The joint becomes red, hot, and swollen due to an acute inflammation.

There are many causes. Seek medical advice as investigations (X-rays, blood tests, etc.) are needed to find the underlying cause. The joint should be rested.

Constitutional treatment from a professional homeopath is required, but the following remedies may give some relief whilst awaiting an appointment. Your homeopath may also recommend nutritional support with vitamins, trace elements, and fish oils.

Take a tablet of the suggested remedy every 15 minutes until there is improvement, then reduce the frequency of the tablets.

• Painful joint without any other signs: RUTA 6C

• Red, hot joint, worse for touch: BELLADONNA 6C and BRYONIA 6C

• Cold, red joint, worse for touch: COLCHICUM 6C

• Extreme swelling of the joint, worse for touch: APIS MELLIFICA 6C

Asthma

Spasm of the small bronchi may be caused by allergy in some cases of asthma. Conventional desensitization to the allergen is not usually helpful. Constitutional homeopathic treatment is required. Your homeopath will advise you on the use of inhalants.

The following remedies may be of use for an acute attack. If improvement does not occur rapidly, or there is any other concern, seek medical advice immediately. Asthma can be life threatening.

For an acute attack, the following remedies are suggested in a dose of one tablet every 15 minutes:

• For all cases: ANTIMONIUM TARTARICUM 6C, IPECAC 6C, and BLATTA ORIENTALIS 6C

Other remedies can be added according to the circumstances:

• Aggravation in damp weather: DULCAMARA 6C

• Intense restlessness and alternation with eczema: ARSENICUM ALBUM 6C

• Worse at bedtime: ARALIA RACEMOSA 6C

• Worse at midnight, with profuse sweating: SAMBUCUS NIGRA 6C

• Worse between 2 and 4 a.m. in a weak person who is very sensitive to the cold: KALI CARBONICUM 6C

• Worse at 3 a.m. in a fat, apathetic person: AMMONIUM CARBONICUM 6C

Athlete's foot

See 'Fungal infections'.

Aversion to food

Aversions to certain types of food are seen in the following remedies. They are part of the remedy picture.

• Aversion to all types of food: COLCHICUM and STANNUM METALLICUM

• Aversion to beer: NUX VOMICA, CHAMOMILLA, CHINA, COCCULUS, NATRUM SULPHURICUM, PHOSPHORUS, and RHUS TOXICODENDRON

• Aversion to bread: CHINA, NATRUM MURIATICUM, CONIUM, KALI CARBONICUM, PULSATILLA, and SEPIA

• Aversion to butter: ARSENICUM ALBUM, PULSATILLA, CARBO VEGETABILIS, NATRUM MURIATICUM, and CHINA

• Aversion to coffee: CALCAREA CARBONICA, BRYONIA, CHINA, COFFEA, DULCAMARA, LYCOPODIUM, NATRUM MURIATICUM, NUX VOMICA, PHOSPHORUS, and SPIGELIA

• Aversion to fatty foods in general: CARBO VEGETABILIS, CYCLAMEN, PULSATILLA, CINA, HEPAR SULPH, PETROLEUM, COLCHICUM, and SEPIA

• Aversion to kitchen smells: COCCULUS, ARSENICUM ALBUM, COLCHICUM, IPECAC, PODOPHYLLUM, and SEPIA

• Aversion to meat: ARSENICUM ALBUM, CHINA, ARNICA, BRYONIA, ALUMINA, CALCAREA CARBONICA, PULSATILLA, and SEPIA

• Aversion to milk: CALCAREA CARBONICA, CALCAREA SULPHURICA, CINA, NATRUM CARBONICUM, LAC DEFLORATUM, NATRUM SULPHURICUM, PULSATILLA, SEPIA, SILICA, and SULPHUR

• Aversion to tobacco: IGNATIA and CALCAREA CARBONICA

Bad breath

See 'The Mouth'.

Baldness

See 'Skin, hair, and nails'.

Bed clothes thrown off

Some people throw off the bedclothes during the night when feverish. This is part of the remedy picture.

• Person looks for a cool spot in the bed: SULPHUR, CHAMOMILLA, PULSATILLA, and SANGUINARIA

• The bedclothes are thrown off during the fever, despite shivering: ACONITE

• The bedclothes are thrown off to relieve pain, as they feel too heavy: APIS MELLIFICA

Bedsores

When a person is confined to bed and their position is not changed frequently, bedsores may result. They are preventable by moving the sick person on a regular basis, and using a special air filled mattress.

• As a preventative, or to heal established sores: ARNICA 6C and LACHESIS 6C taken four times a day whilst the person is bedridden

Bedwetting (enuresis)

After the age of four, involuntary and unconscious emission of urine at night is termed enuresis.

Never blame the child and never use violence. Medical treatment can often prove ineffective.

While awaiting a consultation, give the child a tablet of EQUISETUM HYEMALE 6C morning and night. Add, according to the situation, one tablet of one of the following remedies:

• For enuresis at the beginning of the night in a solitary or unruly child: SEPIA 6C

• When the urine is very dark, with an extremely strong smell: BENZOIC ACID 6C

• For a stubborn, hypersensitive child with sweaty feet: SILICA 6C

• For a child who tosses and turns while asleep and has problems concentrating at school: ZINCUM 6C

Behavioural problems

Temper tantrums and night terrors can disrupt family life. Constitutional remedies are necessary, but minor behavioural problems can be treated at home. Psychological treatment may be needed in some cases. Avoid sedatives and tranquillizing medication if at all possible. It is far better to deal with the underlying problems, rather than masking them with this type of medicine.

Temper tantrums and fits of anger: use one tablet morning and night, and when there is a flare-up of the problem.

• Restless, bad tempered, capricious children: CHAMOMILLA 6C

• Over-worked adults, who express their anger by swearing: ANACARDIUM ORIENTALE 6C

• Hyperactive adults, who are overbearing and are prone to explosive bouts of anger: NUX VOMICA 6C

• Anger leading to neuralgic pains, spasms, and cramps: COLOCYNTHIS 6C

• Suppressed anger in emotionally sensitive individuals, prone to stomach cramps and urinary tract problems: STAPHYSAGRIA 6C

Night terror and nightmares in children

In all cases: HYOSCYMUS 6C and STRAMONIUM 6C after the evening meal. Add as needed:

• CINA 6C if the child is fidgety and suffers with worms (pinworms)

• KALI BROMATUM if there is grinding of the teeth and moaning whilst sleeping

Belching

See abdominal wind under 'Digestive disorders'.

Bites

See 'Trauma and haemorrhages'.

Blepharitis

See 'The eye'.

Blocked nose

This unpleasant symptom often accompanies a head cold, sinusitis, and upper respiratory tract infections.

Take a tablet of one of the following remedies, depending on the situation, every two hours:

• Dry, blocked nose: STICTA PULMONARIA 6C and SAMBUCUS NIGRA 6C

• Nose blocked at night, runny during the day: NUX VOMICA 6C

• Blocked nose with irritating nasal discharge and watery eyes, which are not irritating: ALLIUM CEPA 6C

• Blocked nose with non-irritating discharge, watery eyes with irritation: EUPHRASIA 6C

Boils

See 'Abscesses and boils'.

Homeopathy encyclopedia

Breast-feeding

In the last 20 years, breast-feeding has regained popularity. This natural means of feeding a baby has benefits for the mother, as well as the child. There is no better diet for the baby. Problems may be dealt with using homeopathic remedies as described below.

Problems of the nursing mother

Breast care
Minor irritations of the nipple respond well to bathing the area with diluted CALENDULA tincture (30 drops of the mother tincture in a bowl of warm water). If other problems occur, they must be treated quickly, so have the remedies to hand.

• Sensitive breasts with pain in the breast: ARNICA 6C, CHAMOMILLA 6C, and CROTON TIGLIUM 6C, one tablet of each 15 minutes before each feed

• Swollen breasts (mastitis) with threat of abscess formation: consult your doctor or medical homeopath immediately. Antibiotic therapy may be required

• Cracked nipples without complications: PHYTOLACCA 6C, 15 minutes before each feed

• Cracked nipples with sores: PHYTOLACCA 6C, PETROLEUM 6C, and CASTOR EQUI 6C, one tablet of each 15 minutes before feeding

• Insufficient milk: RICINUS 6C and URTICA URENS 6C, one tablet three times a day

• Excessive milk production (galactorrhoea): PULSATILLA 6C, and LAC CANINUM 6C one tablet of each three times a day

• Excessive fatigue during feeding: CHINA 6C and PHOSPHORIC ACID 6C three times a day

Weaning
Take one dose of PULSATILLA 30C, then CALCAREA CARBONICA 6C and LAC CANINUM 6C three times a day.

Problems of the baby

The baby may suffer from minor problems, such as hiccups, passing excessive wind, sweating during feeding, or minor vomiting. If the vomiting is recurrent, projectile, or excessive, or the baby is unwell in any way, see your doctor as soon as possible. There may be an underlying medical problem.

Breast milk is the best for the baby, but if breast-feeding is not possible your homeopath can recommend remedies to help with the problems of bottle-feeding.

For babies, it is easiest to use granules dissolved in water. If these are not available, crush the tablets between two clean spoons, and then add the powder to water.

• Hiccups: This is caused by a spasmodic contraction of the diaphragm. Give CUPRUM METALLICUM 6C, IGNA-

TIA 6C, and HYOSCYMUS 6C, one granule or tablet of each before feeds

• Belching during and after feeding: ARGENTUM NITRICUM, one granule or tablet before every feed

• The baby falls asleep whilst feeding: OPIUM 15C, one granule or tablet before each feed

• The baby sweats profusely whilst feeding: CALCAREA CARBONICA 6C, one granule or tablet before each feed

• The baby vomits while feeding: AETHUSA CYNAPIUM 6C, one granule or tablet before each feed

Breath, bad

See 'The mouth'.

Breathlessness

See 'Asthma'.

Bronchiolitis

This occurs in small children and causes incessant coughing, difficulty in breathing and congestion in the airways. It requires urgent medical attention and in most cases admission to hospital. Usually, it is a result of a viral infection, but allergy and pollution may be involved. Once the acute illness is over, constitutional homeopathic treatment may prevent further attacks. Whilst waiting for the doctor, you can

give HISTAMINE 6C, BLATTA ORIENTALIS 6C, and IPECAC 6C, one tablet of each every 15 minutes.

Bronchitis

See 'Coughs and bronchitis'.

Bruises

See 'Trauma and burns'.

Bulimia

This is a serious psychological condition that requires professional treatment. Homeopathy can play a part in the therapy.

Comfort eating may be treated with several remedies.

• Almost permanent sensation of hunger, with a desire to eat large quantities of food: ANTIMONIUM CRUDUM 6C twice daily

• Comfort eating following an emotional setback: IGNATIA 6C twice daily

Calculi (stones)

See 'Colic' and 'Diarrhoea'. Calculi, or stones, in the gall bladder or urinary tract require professional homeopathic treatment. Surgery may be required in many cases.

Calluses

See 'Skin, hair, and nails'.

Homeopathy encyclopedia

Calluses

Caries

See 'Teeth'.

Cataract

See 'The eye'

Cellulite

Constitutional homeopathic treatment may help reduce this condition. Your homeopath may prescribe the following remedies: PULSATILLA, NATRUM MURIATICUM, THUJA, NATRUM SULPHURICUM, KALI CARBONICUM, and CALCAREA CARBONICA. Physical exercise, sensible eating habits and reduction of stress will also help.

Drainage remedies to encourage the circulation can be tried: BERBERIS 6C and PAREIRA BRAVA 6C taken twice daily.

Chapped skin

See 'Skin, hair, and nails'.

Character traits

A homeopathic doctor will ask questions in a consultation that may sometimes be surprising. Patients are always asked about their character traits, not in order to modify them through treatment but to get a better idea of which constitutional remedy would be suitable. A few examples are listed below:

- Authoritarian: LYCOPODIUM, AURUM METALLICUM, and NUX VOMICA

- Quick-tempered: CHAMOMILLA, NUX VOMICA and AURUM METALLICUM

- Irritable: NUX VOMICA

- Sullen: NATRUM MURIATICUM

- Capricious: IGNATIA and PULSATILLA

- Impatient: ARGENTUM NITRICUM

- Introverted: STAPHYSAGRIA

- Jealous: LACHESIS

- Shy: PULSATILLA, NATRUM MURIATICUM and SILICA

- Meticulous: ARSENICUM ALBUM

- Hyperactive and optimistic: SULPHUR

- Very emotional: GELSEMIUM and IGNATIA

Chicken pox

See 'Childhood illnesses'.

Childbirth

Childbirth is a natural process, which is usually trouble free. Homeopathic remedies work wonderfully during pregnancy, and can improve contractions in labour and dispel the fears of the mother-to-be.

Seek professional advice as remedies are used in different potencies during pregnancy.

Your homeopath may suggest the following remedies:

• CAULOPHYLLUM – for labour to run smoothly

• ARNICA – to reduce bruising in childbirth

• CHINA – for the blood and fluid loss in labour

• CIMICIFUGA – for fear of labour

• GELSEMIUM – for fear of labour

Please note that remedies cannot help if the baby is in an unfavourable position such as breech presentation, or if the pelvis is too small for a normal delivery. Homeopathy can assist with recovery from a Caesarean section.

Childhood illnesses

Scarlet fever, measles, Rubella (German measles), and chicken pox present with fever and skin rashes. Scarlet fever is fortunately rare nowadays, as it can be serious if it affects the kidneys.

Consult your doctor to make the diagnosis. While you are waiting, you can start the appropriate treatment from the following.

Scarlet fever

Scarlet fever is caused by the Streptococcus bacterium, which can be very damaging to the kidneys. It is not suitable for self-medication. Treatment will usually require antibiotics.

Mumps

This is a viral infection of the parotid salivary glands located behind the ear; it is almost always benign in children.

At the start, three remedies are indicated: ACONITE 6C, BELLADONNA 6C, and FERRUM PHOSPHORICUM 6C, one tablet of each, four times a day. When the parotids swell, replace ACONITE with MERCURIUS VIVUS 6C. During convalescence from mumps, take PULSATILLA 6C and SULPHUR IODATUM 6C, one tablet in the morning and evening for a week.

Measles

At the start, give ACONITE 6C, BELLADONNA 6C, and FERRUM PHOSPHORICUM 6C, one tablet of each, four times a day, then decrease the frequency of the remedies when you notice an improvement. If necessary add:

• when a dry, troublesome cough appears: BRYONIA 6C

• when a child is thirstless and shaky: GELSEMIUM 6C

• when there is a runny nose and watery eyes: ALLIUM CEPA 6C and EUPHRASIA 6C

Homeopathy encyclopedia

• when there is a very red throat with white spots and 'furred' tongue: MERCURIUS VIVUS 6C

• when the rash appears: PULSATILLA 6C

During convalescence from mumps give PULSATILLA 6C and SULPHUR IODATUM 6C, one tablet in the morning and evening for a week.

Rubella (German measles)

This disease is serious in pregnant women as it can cause deformities in the unborn child. If your child develops it, ensure he or she stays indoors and no pregnant women visit.

At the start, three remedies are indicated: ACONITE 6C, BELLADONNA 6C, and FERRUM PHOSPHORICUM 6C, one tablet of each, four times a day, decreasing the frequency when you notice an improvement. When spots are appearing give PULSATILLA 6C.

During convalescence from Rubella, give PULSATILLA 6C and SULPHUR IODATUM 6C, one tablet in the morning and evening for a week.

Chicken pox

Chicken pox may recur in later life when the immunity is low as shingles.

At the start, three remedies are indicated: ACONITE 6C, BELLADONNA 6C, and FERRUM PHOSPHORICUM 6C, one tablet of each, four times a day, decreasing the frequency, when you notice an improvement.

• When the spots (fluid containing blisters) are appearing, give RHUS TOXICODENDRON 6C four times a day

• When the blisters become irritated and scabs appear, replace RHUS TOXICODENDRON with MEZERIUM 6C and MERCURIUS VIVUS 6C, one tablet of each four times a day

During convalescence, give PULSATILLA 6C, and SULPHUR IODATUM 6C, one tablet of each in the morning and evening for a week.

Chill

At the first appearance of symptoms following a cold snap, take one tablet every two hours of ACONITE 6C, FERRUM PHOSPHORICUM 6C, and BELLADONNA 6C.

Cholecystitis

An acute inflammation of the gall bladder always requires medical intervention. While awaiting treatment, put an ice pack on the patient's stomach and give a tablet of each of the following every 15 minutes: COLOCYNTHIS 6C, BELLADONNA 6C, and BRYONIA 6C.

Cholesterol

An elevated blood cholesterol level requires a full medical check-up and professional homeopathic treatment. If left untreated it may lead to atherosclerosis.

A change of diet to the Mediterranean-style diet may help. As lipid-lowering drugs can cause many side effects, your homeopath will prescribe a constitutional remedy, such as LYCOPODIUM, NUX VOMICA, SEPIA, or SULPHUR, to assist the body to rebalance the cholesterol levels.

Coffee

Coffee is more toxic than one would expect. It can aggravate inflammatory conditions and the pain of osteoarthritis, as well as causing palpitations, diarrhoea, headaches, and insomnia. To combat the toxicity of excessive coffee drinking, stop coffee and detoxify with NUX VOMICA 6C, THUJA 6C, and COFFEA 6C, one tablet of each twice daily.

There are various reactions to coffee that may assist in choosing a constitutional remedy.

• Aversion to coffee: CALCAREA CARBONICA

• Aggravation of a condition brought on by drinking coffee: COFFEA

• Craving for coffee: NUX VOMICA

• Diarrhoea after drinking coffee: ALOE SOCOTRINA

Cold sores

See 'Herpes'

Colds

A wide range of viruses called 'rhinoviruses' cause the common cold, with a runny nose and congestion in the head.

Keep warm and avoid cold cures from the chemist as these only suppress the symptoms.

As soon as the first symptoms appear, take one tablet every 15 minutes, decreasing the frequency when an improvement is noted, of ALLIUM CEPA 6C, EUPHRASIA 6C, and FERRUM PHOSPHORICUM 6C. Add one of the following, according to the situation:

– If fever is present and the throat is dry and red: BELLADONNA 6C

– With sneezing and a feeling of intense cold: CAMPHORA 6C

– With abundant secretion and pains at the root of the nose: KALI IODATUM 6C

– When the nose is runny by day but blocked at night: NUX VOMICA 6C

– When there are greenish-yellow scabs blocking the nose: KALI BICHROMICUM 6C

– When the nose is totally blocked with a pinching feeling at the root of the nose: STICTA PULMONARIA 6C

If you catch colds very frequently, consider looking for an underlying allergic cause. Avoid using nose drops that

Homeopathy encyclopedia

temporarily unblock the nose but later aggravate the symptoms.

Colic

Gall-bladder colic

This painful spasm can be caused by a stone or sludge in the gall bladder. It may come on after eating a fatty meal. If fever or jaundice is present, see your doctor immediately. Even without these symptoms, a full medical examination and investigations should be performed.

To ease the pain, the following remedies may be useful: BERBERIS VULGARIS 6C, CHELEDONIUM 6C, CHINA 6C, PULSATILLA 6C, and IGNATIA 6C, one tablet of each taken every 15 minutes. As soon as there is improvement, reduce the frequency of the remedies.

Kidney colic

A stone in the urinary tract can cause severe pain. Surgery is often required to remove the stone. Certain remedies may ease the pain whilst awaiting an urgent medical assessment: BELLADONNA 6C, CALCAREA CARBONICA 6C, LYCOPODIUM 6C, and PRAVEIRA BRAVA 6C taken every 15 minutes.

Comfort eating

See 'Bulimia'.

Conjunctivitis

See 'The Eye'.

Consolation and comforting

A person's reaction to being comforted or consoled can be useful in deciding on a constitutional remedy.

• A person who cries easily and feels better after consolation: PULSATILLA

• Isolated, introverted person, worse from consolation: NATRUM MURIATICUM

• An indecisive, weak person irritated by fussing and consolation: SILICA

• A person aggravated by consolation but improved by distractions: IGNATIA

Constipation

Constipation has many causes. Any recent alteration in bowel habit should be fully investigated, especially if blood or mucus is passed, as it may be a sign of underlying disease in the bowel.

Laxatives should be avoided if possible as they cause irritation of the intestines.

Homeopathic remedies may be very useful in treating constipation. Try a dose of one of the following morning and night:

• No desire to open the bowels, very hard stools that are large or in small pieces: BRYONIA ALBA 6C

• No desire to open the bowels, great strain needed to pass a normal stool: ALUMINA 6C

• No desire to open the bowels for several days, large, hard stool with mucus: GRAPHITES 6C

• Frequent desire to open the bowels, without adequate result. Impression of incomplete evacuation: LYCOPODIUM 6C

• Pain during bowel movements in a dehydrated person: NATRUM MURIATICUM 6C

• Frequent need for bowel movements but all attempts fruitless in an irritable and overbearing person: NUX VOMICA 6C

• Constipation after travelling or change of routine: PLATINA 6C

• Total inertia of the bowel with dry, black stools, often after an operation: OPIUM 6C

• Constipation in a person with gallbladder or liver disease: CHELEDONIUM 6C

• Incomplete evacuation with abdominal bloating in a person with liver disease: HYDRASTIS 6C

• Constipation in the elderly: CAUSTICUM 6C

Convalescence

Following any serious illness, operation or accident, the body is fragile and needs to convalesce. Take SULPHUR IODATUM 6C and MANGANUM 6C twice daily, in addition to a constitutional remedy.

Corns

Corns on the feet often recur after they have been removed. To solve the problem take: LYCOPODIUM 6C, ANTIMONIUM CRUDUM 6C and THUJA 6C twice daily for several weeks.

Coughs and bronchitis

A cough is a reflex action to expel air in the lungs forcibly following irritation in the air passages. Bronchitis is an inflammation of the bronchi (main air passages) and is often infectious. It is accompanied by a cough and, in many cases, a fever.

A cough is merely a symptom. Persistent coughs need investigation. Coughing up blood needs urgent medical attention.

Coughs following colds can be treated at home.

Homeopathy encyclopedia

Dry cough (without expectoration)

• Combined with infections of the nose, pharynx, and sinuses: take one tablet of each of the following four times a day, BELLADONNA 6C, NUX VOMICA 6C, and SANGUINARIA 6C

• Combined with laryngitis: take one of each of the following four times a day, ACONITE 6C, SPONGIA TOSTA 6C, and SAMBUCUS NIGRA 6C

• Combined with infections of the trachea (tracheitis): take one tablet of RUMEX CRISPUS 6C and STICTA PULMONARIA 6C four times a day

• Combined with infections of the trachea and bronchi: take BRYONIA ALBA 6C four times a day and HEPAR SULPH 30C every other day

Irritating coughs

• Take one tablet of the chosen remedy four times a day and at the start of a coughing bout

• Before there is any phlegm: DROSERA 6C

• With abundant clear, sticky phlegm: COCCUS CACTI 6C

• With nausea, unrelieved by vomiting: IPECAC 6C

• Incessant coughing, with spasms of the throat: CUPRUM METALLICUM 6C

Productive cough

In all cases, take one tablet of FERRUM PHOSPHORICUM 6C and HEPAR SULPH 6C four times a day, plus one of the following:

• Painful cough with thick yellow phlegm: KALI BICHROMICUM 6C

• Cough with green phlegm and foul mucus: MERCURIUS VIVUS 6C

• Loose cough with yellow phlegm during the day, dry cough at night: PULSATILLA 6C

• Cough brought on or made worse by damp weather: DULCAMARA 6C

• Chronic cough with foul phlegm: SILICA 6C

• Cough with nausea, unrelieved by vomiting: IPECAC 6C

• Cough with phlegm that is difficult to bring up: ANTIMONIUM TARTARICUM 6C

Bronchitis

This requires medical attention if there is no improvement within 24 hours.

In all cases take HEPAR SULPH 30C twice daily and one tablet of each of the following four times a day: ANTIMONIUM TARTARICUM 6C, IPECAC 6C, and BRYONIA 6C.

Add one of the following as necessary:

• MERCURIUS VIVUS 6C for large lumps of yellow phlegm

• KALI BICHROMIUM 6C for green, loose phlegm.

Looking after yourself

Cramps

These painful, involuntary muscle spasms may occur after unaccustomed exercise or at rest in bed at night. Take one tablet of each of the following twice a day, and during the episodes of cramp: CUPRUM METALLICUM 6C, MAGNESIA PHOSHORICA 6C, and NUX VOMICA 6C.

Cravings

Your homeopath will take note of food cravings, which will assist on deciding on a constitutional remedy:

• Acidic foods: SEPIA, NATRUM MURIATICUM, and ANTIMONIUM CRUDUM

• Alcohol: SULPHUR, LACHESIS, NUX VOMICA, CONIUM, and CAPSICUM

• Beer: KALI BICHROMICUM, ALOE, NUX VOMICA, SULPHUR, CAUSTICUM, and PSORINUM

• Bread: MAGNESIA CARBONICA, NATRUM MURIATICUM, ARSENICUM ALBUM, and FERRUM PHOSPHORICUM

• Butter: MERCURIUS VIVIUS and FERRUM PHOSPHORICUM

• Coffee: NUX VOMICA, ANGUSTURA, AURUM METALLICUM, CHAMOMILLA, NUX MOSCHATA, and CARBO VEGETABILIS

• Fatty foods: SULPHUR, NUX VOMICA, and NITRIC ACID

• Fish: NATRUM MURIATICUM

• Fizzy drinks: CHINA, LYCOPODIUM, CARBO VEGETABILIS, and KALI CARBONICUM

• Fruit: MAGNESIA CARBONICA, PHOSPHORIC ACID, VERATRUM ALBUM, CHINA, SULPHURIC ACID, and ANTIMONIUM TARTARICUM

• Hot drinks: ARSENICUM ALBUM, LYCOPODIUM, SABADILLA, EUPATORIUM, and MEDORRHINUM

• Hot food: LYCOPODIUM, CHELEDONIUM, and ARSENICUM ALBUM

• Ice cream: CALCAREA CARBONICA, PHOSPHORUS, and VERATRUM ALBUM

• Indigestible foods: CALCAREA CARBONICA, CALCAREA PHOSPHORICA, and ALUMINA

• Meat: ALLIUM SATIVA, MAGNESIA CARBONICA, and CALCAREA PHOSPHORICA

• Milk: ABROTANUM, PHOSPHORIC ACID, and STAPHYSAGRIA

• Oysters: LACHESIS, CALCAREA CARBONICA, and NATRUM MURIATICUM

• Salty food: NATRUM MURIATICUM, CALCAREA PHOSPHORICA, CARBO VEGETABILIS, PHOSPHORUS, and ARGENTUM NITRICUM

• Smoked meats: CALCAREA PHOSPHORICA and CAUSTICUM

Homeopathy encyclopedia

• Spicy foods: SEPIA, NUX VOMICA, NATRUM MURIATICUM, HEPAR SULPH, SULPHUR, and PHOSPHORUS

• Sugar: CHINA, LYCOPODIUM, ARGENTUM NITRICUM, KALI CARBONICUM, SULPHUR, CALCAREA CARBONICA, CARBO VEGETABILIS, and NATRUM CARBONICUM

See also 'Overeating'.

Cuts

See 'Trauma and burns'.

Cyst

A cyst is a benign tumour, which is often soft to the touch. It can occur anywhere on the body. It is important to consult a doctor to make the diagnosis. Homeopathic treatment may be helpful in stopping it growing, or in some cases reducing its size.

Cystitis

If the urine is clear and there are no obvious signs of a urinary tract infection (cloudy, offensive urine and fever) STAPHYSAGRIA 6C twice daily can ease the discomfort whilst passing urine. Drink plenty of water as this will help flush out any bacteria.

Homeopathic remedies can help in urinary infections, but if fever is present or there is blood in the urine see your doctor as soon as possible. Recurrent infections need investigating. If symptoms do not settle within 24 hours or you are unwell with fever, severe pain, or vomiting, consult your doctor.

As soon as the symptoms occur, start taking the remedies every 15 minutes until there is improvement, then reduce the frequency of the tablets: CANTHARIS 6C, MERCURIUS CORROSIVUS 6C, and FORMICA RUFA 6C.

Death, fear of

A person can be fearful of death during an acute illness, or have a longstanding fear. Certain remedies can help calm the person.

• Panic and fear of imminent death: ACONITE 30C, one tablet every ten minutes until everything is back to normal

• Fear of death because of chronic disease: AURUM, ARSENICUM ALBUM, AGNUS CASTUS, PSORINUM, PHOSPHORUS, and MEDORRHINUM

Choose the remedy on the basis of the patient's personality.

Decalcification

See also 'Osteoporosis' under 'Menopause'.

To improve the assimilation and consolidation of calcium: CALCAREA PHOSPHORICA 6C and SYMPHYTUM 6C, one tablet in the morning and evening, and SILICA 6C daily for two to three months.

Dehydration

Infants with severe diarrhoea are in danger of dehydration. Urgent medical attention is therefore required and this may lead to admission to hospital to evaluate the extent of water loss, look for the causes, and start treatment.

While waiting for the doctor, administer one granule or tablet of PODOPHYL-LUM 6C and VERATRUM ALBUM 6C every 30 minutes.

Once the acute episode is over, homeopathic treatment will help the recovery process. Administer MANGANUM 6C and CHINA 6C, one tablet of each three times a day for two months.

Delirium

Delirium is a mental disorder characterized by hallucinations that contradict reality and are impervious to criticism. It can occur in illnesses, especially where fever is present. Consult your doctor urgently with any such disorder. Homeopathy may complement medical treatment, but only under the supervision of a professional homeopath, who may suggest the following remedies:

• Furious, violent delirium with aggression: HYOSCYMUS or STRAMONIUM.

• Delirium with hallucinations and great loquacity (often found in alcoholics): LACHESIS

• Delirium with high fever: BELLADONNA

• Calm delirium with pale face and physical restlessness: RHUS TOXICODENDRON

Depression

A homeopath is generally needed to treat depression, as it requires a careful choice of constitutional remedies and potency. Self-medication can, however, obtain results, especially at the start of the sickness, but it is difficult to choose the right remedy and potency. Contact the doctor immediately if there is any suicidal intent.

In all cases, use the high dilutions of 30C, at a rate of one tablet in the morning and evening. If there is no rapid response (within a week), consult your doctor or homeopath. The following remedies may be helpful:

• After setbacks, sadness, or mourning: STAPHYSAGRIA and IGNATIA

• Anxious and depressed person, who fears he or she will never be cured: ARSENICUM ALBUM

• Disgust with life in a pessimistic person: AURUM METALLICUM

• Following intellectual overexertion, with memory problems: KALI PHOSPHORICUM

• Solitary person who constantly broods, and refuses consolation: NATRUM MURIATICUM

• Post-natal depression: SEPIA

• Hypersensitive, inhibited person: AMBRA GRISEA, IGNATIA

• Menopausal depression: LACHESIS

• Tired person who becomes indifferent to everything: PHOSPHORIC ACID

Warning

Always avoid stimulants (including tea and coffee) that only mask tiredness and depression, and will lead to exhaustion.

Desensitization

Desensitization, by means of intra-dermal injections of increasing doses of an allergen (sensitizing substance) has long been considered an excellent method for curing an allergy. Years of practice, however, have led to countless failures using this approach.

The homeopathic technique, which as always uses very weak dilutions and, moreover, decreasing doses, obtains far better results.

MIXED POLLENS AND GRASSES 30C taken weekly is an excellent remedy for hay fever.

Homeopathy is sometimes needed to cure the side effects (red skin and swelling) of traditional desensitization. In

these cases, use: APIS MELLIFICA 6C and HISTAMINE 6C, one tablet of each, three times a day, while the problems persist.

Diabetes

Diabetes is often hereditary, and leads to high blood sugar as well as elevated cholesterol and triglyceride levels. It affects many of the organs of the body: the heart and blood vessels, the kidneys, and the eyes. Medication, in the form of tablets or insulin injections, may be recommended in addition to a strict diet.

Homeopathic remedies are excellent complements to a classical treatment but they can only be chosen by a homeopath.

Diarrhoea

For all types of diarrhoea: PODOPHYL-LUM 6C, one tablet every two hours, reducing the frequency of the remedy when you notice an improvement. Add one tablet of the chosen remedy every two hours, depending on the symptoms:

• With burning, foul-smelling stools, fever, and an infectious condition (or food poisoning): ARSENICUM ALBUM 6C

• Very abundant stools with great weakness and cold sweating, or after excessive consumption of fruit: VERATRUM ALBUM 6C

• Green stools after excessive consumption of sugar: ARGENTUM NITRICUM 6C

• Half-solid and half-liquid stools after overeating: ANTIMONIUM CRUDUM 6C

• Stools expelled early in the morning in a jet, with a great deal of wind: NATRUM SULPHURICUM 6C

• Very liquid stools, almost like water, with no pain, but leaving the person exhausted: CHINA 6C

• Colourless, white stools, leaving a very tired person exhausted: PHOSPHORIC ACID 6C

• Stools which cannot be held in and are expelled immediately after eating or drinking: ALOE SOCOTRINA 6C

• Stools producing pains that are improved by doubling over, with the knees against the chest: COLOCYNTHIS 6C

• Burning stools with vomiting of bile: IRIS VESICOLOR 6C

• During periods: VERATRUM ALBUM 6C

• After excessive consumption of fatty foods or ice cream: PULSATILLA 6C

• After excessive consumption of alcohol: NUX VOMICA 6C

• After eating oysters: LYCOPODIUM 6C and ARSENICUM ALBUM 6C

• After excessive consumption of milk or dairy products: MAGNESIA MURIATICA 6C

• After excitement (good or bad news): GELSEMIUM 6C

Traveller's diarrhoea

This type of diarrhoea is food-related and afflicts 30 to 50 per cent of travellers visiting the tropics. The number of bowel movements each day can vary greatly and is often considerable (10 to 20!).

The strict application of the Law of Similars makes it possible to select effective homeopathic remedies and produces remarkable results. However, such remedies are rare in the tropics. You must therefore consider taking them all with you – and that is a lot of medicines!

The use of classical medicines prescribed by your doctor will enable you to solve the problem.

Diet

Homeopaths ask numerous questions about eating habits, not only in connection with excess body weight but also as an aid to prescribing constitutional remedies. It is therefore very important to provide as much information as possible about your craving for or aversion to different foodstuffs.

See also 'Obesity'.

Digestive disorders

For Mediterranean diet see 'Arteriosclerosis'.

Digestive disorders

Abdominal bloating, pain, heartburn, and vomiting are the most common disorders of the digestive system, and they may have a psychological cause. If the symptoms are long-standing or recurrent, see your doctor to exclude any underlying disease.

Improve your diet, increase your physical activity, and reduce stress.

Abdominal bloating

Some digestive problems create a feeling of excessive air in the stomach or intestines. These are most often due to poor diet or emotional upset.

Depending on the situation, take one tablet of the following remedies every 30 minutes:

• With sleepiness after eating a meal, in a nervous and impatient person, who has a large appetite: NUX VOMICA 6C

• During menstrual periods: COCCULUS INDICIS 6C

• With urgent, burning diarrhoea: ALOE SOCOTRINA 6C

• When triggered by fatty food and improved by fizzy drinks: CARBO VEGETABILIS 6C

• When the stomach is extremely bloated and everything seems to turn into gas: CARBO VEGETABILIS 6C

• With noisy burping in a very anxious subject: ARGENTUM NITRICUM 6C

• When triggered by an emotional setback, even without having eaten: IGNATIA 6C

• When triggered by fruit and vegetables, with a tendency to diarrhoea: CHINA 6C

• With a feeling of fullness immediately after eating in a person suffering from a liver complaint: LYCOPODIUM 6C

• With constant rumbling: THUJA 6C

Abdominal pain

Start with the combination of COLOCYNTHIS 6C, MAGNESIA PHOSPHORICA 6C, CUPRUM 6C, and LYCOPODIUM 6C, taking a tablet of each every 15 minutes, reducing the frequency as improvement occurs. Then add one tablet of the chosen remedy every two hours:

• Abdominal pain with fever: BELLADONNA 6C

• Abdominal pain improved by stretching: DIOSCOREA 6C

• Abdominal pain after a cold snap: ACONITE 6C

• Abdominal pain after an emotional setback: IGNATIA 6C

• Abdominal pain with heartburn or

Looking after yourself

excess acidity: ROBINA 6C and SUPHURIC ACID 6C

• Abdominal cramps: NUX VOMICA 6C and MAGNESIA PHOSPHORICA 6C

• Abdominal pain with indigestion: NUX VOMICA 6C

Abdominal wind (belching, flatulence)

Take one tablet of the following remedies every hour: IGNATIA 6C, ARGENTUM NITRICUM 6C, and NUX VOMICA 6C. Add one of these remedies if needed:

• For a swollen stomach relieved by passing wind: CARBO VEGETABILIS 6C

• If belching does not bring relief: CHINA 6C

• If belching is very frequent: ASA FOETIDA 6C

• When all food seems to produce wind: KALI CARBONICUM 6C

Heartburn or acidity in the stomach

Two remedies, IRIS VESICOLOR 6C and ROBINA 6C, one tablet in the morning and evening and whenever there is a flare up, can soothe acidic burning in the stomach with belching, excessive salivation, nausea, and, at times, vomiting.

• If the burning is accompanied by intolerance of dairy products, add MAGNESIA CARBONICA 6C, one tablet whenever the problem occurs.

• If the burning is accompanied by

cramps and improved by drinking something cold, add CURPRUM METALLICUM 6C, one tablet whenever the problem occurs

Hiatus hernia

This term is used when part of the stomach rises up through the diaphragm at the opening to the oesophagus (gullet). The resulting pains are appeased by ARGENTUM NITRICUM 6C, one tablet in the morning and evening, for a few weeks whilst pain is present. Surgery is rarely required.

Hiccup

A spasmodic contraction of the diaphragm that responds well to these homeopathic remedies: CUPRUM METALLICUM 6C, IGNATIA 6C, and HYOSCYMUS 6C, one tablet of each every two hours.

Stomach ulcer

In addition to the ulcer healing medication prescribed by your doctor, take ARGENTUM NITRICUM 6C and KALI BICHROMIUM 6C twice daily. If the bacterium Helicobacter pylori is present, the doctor will also prescribe a course of antibiotics. Constitutional homeopathic treatment is very helpful in ulcer disease.

Vomiting

If this does not settle rapidly with the chosen remedy, seek medical attention.

In the meantime, take one tablet of the chosen remedy hourly:

• After overindulgence (large meal washed down with lots of alcohol), often with a 'furred' tongue: NUX VOMICA 6C and ANTIMONIUM CRUDUM 6C

• After eating cakes and fatty foods: PULSATILLA 6C

• During teething: CHAMOMILLA 6C

• Vomiting of bile: IRIS VESICOLOR 6C and BRYONIA ALBA 6C

• Violent, foul-smelling vomiting with putrid diarrhoea: ARSENICUM ALBUM 6C

• Constant diarrhoea, and nausea unrelieved by vomiting. The tongue is clean: IPECAC 6C

• In babies during breast-feeding: AETHUSA CYNAPIUM 6C, one crushed tablet before every feed.

Disappointment

A profound feeling of disappointment can be a guide to a suitable remedy.

• Disappointed, bitter, indignant, feeling frustrated and unfairly treated: STAPHYSAGRIA

• Disappointed, frustrated, and constantly brooding over the same things: THUJA.

• Disappointed in love, usually by infidelity: NATRUM MURIATICUM

• Disappointed, irritable, surly, and emotionally sensitive: SILICA

Diuretics

There are no diuretic remedies, in the classical sense of being medicines that stimulate urination very soon after taking them.

However, some remedies do assist the function of the kidneys, as well as easing the pains of kidney colic and helping to pass small stones or gravel. Your homeopath will decide on an appropriate remedy. Useful remedies include:

• PAREIRA BRAVA, when the pain is relieved by the subject doubling up with the knees against the chest.

• BERBERIS VULGARIS, when the pain spreads out in all directions.

• COLOCYNTHIS, if the spasms of pain are relieved when the subject is doubled up

• CHAMOMILLA, when intolerable pain is relieved by moving about briskly.

• CALCAREA CARBONICA, which sometimes acts rapidly on pain.

Diverticulitis

In this condition, the intestinal lining protrudes through the muscular wall of the bowel. The diagnosis of diverticulitis is made after a series of X-rays using a contrast medium (barium enema). A diet and constitutional treatment will help with the symptoms of altered bowel habit and abdominal discomfort. To avoid abdominal pain from a flare up, take MAGNESIA PHOSPHORICA 6C and COLOCYNTHIS 6C, one tablet of each in the morning and evening.

Double vision (diplopia)

Double vision requires an immediate consultation with an ophthalmologist.

If the visual disturbance appears during a migraine, try GELSEMIUM 6C, and CYCLAMEN 6C, one tablet every hour.

Drainage remedies

The concept of drainage remedies dates back to a time when there was great concern about toxins in the food and from atmospheric pollution. Some remedies that were particularly active on our organs of excretion (the lungs, kidneys, skin, and liver) were therefore considered ideal for detoxification.

The concept of toxins has fallen into disuse but 'drainage remedies' are still excellent products for regulating the function of certain organs.

• SOLIDAGO acts on the liver

• SULPHUR IODATUM acts on the skin

• BERBERIS VULGARIS acts on the kidneys

• NUX VOMICA acts on the digestive system

Some homeopaths use these drainage remedies.

Drug tests on athletes

Homeopathic medicines will not give a positive result in a doping test. This undoubtedly explains the growing interest in homeopathy among sports competitors.

The products most widely used to help recovery from vigorous training are ARNICA, RHUS TOXICODENDRON, RUTA, LACTIC ACID, and CUPRUM METALLICUM.

Drunkenness

See 'Alcohol abuse'.

Dry skin or mucous membranes

Dry skin or mucous membranes are common symptoms that usually indicate a more general ailment. While waiting to consult a homeopath, take:

• For dry skin: ALUMINA 6C, ARSENICUM ALBUM 6C, and PETROLEUM 6C, one tablet of each three times a day

• Dry mucous membranes without

thirst: ALUMINA 6C and NUX MOSCHATA 6C, one tablet of each three times a day

• Dry mucous membranes with thirst: BELLADONNA 6C and BRYONIA 6C, one tablet of each three times a day

• Vaginal dryness: ALUMINA 6C, BELLADONNA 6C, and NATRUM MURIATICUM 6C, one tablet of each three times a day, and FOLLICULINUM 30C twice a week

Dyspareunia (pain on sexual intercourse)

This disorder always requires a gynaecological consultation to discover the causes – vaginal dryness (premenopause or menopause), infections, psychological problems – and decide on a treatment.

Your homeopath will be able to complement treatment with remedies.

Ear infections

Ear infections are often treated with antibiotics, although homeopathic remedies can always be tried first.

Do not put anything in your ear unless a doctor tells you to. Drops can be dangerous when the eardrum has been perforated.

At the onset, take ACONITE 6C, FERRUM PHOSPHORICUM 76C, and BELLADONNA 6C, one tablet of each four times a day.

After 24 to 48 hours of the course of the illness, stop ACONITE and add CAPSICUM 6C and ARSENICUM ALBUM 6C, one tablet of each four times a day.

Warning
Recurrent ear infections can damage hearing. They must be treated with constitutional remedies chosen by a homeopath.

Eating disorders

Consult your doctor if the eating disorder persisits.

• Reduced appetite with a desire for salty food, constant thirst, and irritability: NATRUM MURIATICUM 6C, one tablet morning and night

• Reduced appetite with an aversion to fatty foods: PULSATILLA 6C, one tablet morning and night

• Excessive appetite for all kinds of food: ANTIMONIUM CRUDUM 6C, one tablet morning and night

• Excessive appetite with irritability, improved by eating food: ANACARDIUM 6C, one tablet morning and night

• Ravenous hunger triggered by strong

emotions: IGNATIA 6C, one granule morning and night

Eczema

See 'Skin, hair, and nails'.

Emotional problems

See 'Nerves, fear and anxiety'.

Epilepsy

Epilepsy is a serious condition; in many cases the cause is unknown.

Self-medication is out of the question. However, expertly prescribed homeopathic treatment often enhances conventional treatment.

Erection, problems with

See 'Sexual problems'.

Exams, fear of

See 'Nerves, fear, and anxiety'.

Exostosis (heel spurs)

Abnormal bony outgrowths may be seen on X-ray. They are often tender to the touch, and cause recurrent blistering on the heel where they rub against shoes. Some can be felt through the

skin. It is advisable to consult a homeopath. Meanwhile, take HECLA LAVA 6C and CALCAREA FLUORICA 6C, one tablet twice a day.

The eye

The eye can be affected by a number of specific diseases, as well as systemic diseases.

Any serious eye condition is the domain of an eye specialist (ophthalmologist), who must be consulted without hesitation.

Self-medication is safe as long as the vision is unaffected by the condition. If there is no rapid improvement with the homeopathic remedies, contact your doctor.

Take the remedies according to the situation:

• Blepharitis (inflammation of the edge of the eyelids): PULSATILLA 6C, GRAPHITES 6C, and STAPHYSAGRIA 6C, one tablet four times a day, for ten days

• Conjunctivitis: APIS MELLIFICA 6C, BELLADONNA 6C, EUPHRASIA 6C, one tablet four times a day for ten days

• Eyelids stuck together in the morning: PULSATILLA 6C, MERCURIUS VIVUS 6C, GRAPHITES 6C, one tablet four times a day, for ten days

• Stye (small boil on the edge of the eyelid): PULSATILLA 6C and HEPAR

The eye

SULPH 6C, one tablet four times a day, for ten days

• Black eye with normal vision: LEDUM PALUSTRE 6C, one tablet in the morning and evening, for one month

• Watery eyes: EUPHRASIA 6C, ALLIUM CEPA 6C, and PULSATILLA 6C, one tablet four times a day, for ten days

Have regular eye checks at the opticians, wear sunglasses when necessary and, if you wear contact lenses, be strict about hygiene.

Eye strain

Eye strain can occur in tired or overworked people, particularly if they use the computer a lot. Take this combination: ARNICA 6C, HAMAMELIS 6C, and RUTA 6C, one tablet of each four times a day, and reduce any work that strains the eyes.

If the problems persist, consult an ophthalmologist.

Faecal impaction

Accumulation of dry, hard stools may gradually block the rectum; this is particularly found in malnourished, constipated elderly people. A manual evacuation performed by a nurse is often required.

A healthy diet may prevent problems. It should contain lots of roughage in the form of fruit and vegetables, and three to four pints of water a day. Three homeopathic remedies are also useful: OPIUM 6C, ALUMINA 6C, and BRYONIA 6C, one tablet of each three times a day.

Faecal incontinence

A doctor must be consulted if this symptom persists beyond the age of four.

Fainting

Certain individuals feel faint regularly, but rarely actually pass out. Strong emotions evoke this response. Always see your doctor to ensure this is simple fainting, and not something more sinister. Constitutional homeopathic remedies will help prevent further attacks.

Keep calm and make the subject lie down to prevent any injuries caused by falling over.

When the person starts to feel faint, give a tablet of the chosen remedy every 15 minutes:

• For fainting without any obvious cause, prompted by an insignificant event: MOSCHUS 6C

• Following a temper fit or violent emotion: GELSEMIUM 6C

• Following an emotional setback or disappointment: IGNATIA 6C

• During periods: SEPIA 6C

• Following minor blood loss: CHINA 6C

• After a meal with excessive alcohol: NUX VOMICA 6C

• Due to heat in a room: PULSATILLA 6C

• Following exposure to the sun: GLONOINE 6C and APIS MELLIFICA 6C

Fasting

Fasting is not practised much in the West but it is probably one of the best ways of staying in good health. Do not undertake long fasts without expert medical advice. A day or two without eating can be beneficial. When reintroducing food after the fast, ensure that it is light on the stomach and in small quantities initially.

To assist with detoxification, drink plenty of water and use 'drainage remedies' to further cleanse the system. Take BERBERIS VULGARIS 6C, SOLIDAGO 6C, and CHELEDONIUM 6C, one tablet of each, twice a day during the fast and for the week afterwards.

Fatigue

Fatigue is a symptom, not a disease. It may be a signal that you are not taking care of yourself. It can lead to physical and intellectual exhaustion, as well as problems with concentration and

sleeping. It is important to look closely at your lifestyle, and make adjustments to it. Improving your diet and sleeping patterns may be helpful.

Fatigue is normal for a short time following an illness, but if it persists for longer than expected, or there is no obvious cause, consult your doctor.

While awaiting a consultation or the results of tests:

Fatigue in adults

Take MANGANUM 6C each morning.

Add the following remedies, one tablet, morning and night, according to the situation:

• After excessive physical exertion, playing sport or a trauma: ARNICA 6C and RHUS TOXICODENDRON 6C

• In a growing adolescent: CALCAREA PHOSPHORICA 6C

• After fluid loss (diarrhea, vomiting, sweating, heavy periods, and haemorrhage): CHINA 6C

• If fatigue is psychological: KALI PHOSPHORICUM 6C

• After giving birth: SEPIA 6C

• After great emotion, particularly if it is not expressed: GELSEMIUM 6C and STAPHYSAGRIA 6C

Fatigue in schoolchildren

AETHUSA CYNAPIUM 6C, CALCAREA

PHOSPHORICA 6C, and KALI PHOS-PHORICUM 6C, one tablet morning and night for two weeks. If there is no improvement, see the doctor.

Warning
Fatigue can be a symptom of under-lying disease. Consult your doctor if there is any doubt as to the cause.

Fear

See 'Nerves, fear, and anxiety'.

Female reproductive system

Pain and swelling in the breasts, pelvic pain, and vaginal discharge are the most common symptoms found in the female menstrual cycle.

Most of these problems are benign and the homeopathic treatment often deals with them effectively.

Pelvic pain

Pains in the ovaries can have several causes and require a medical consulta-tion. Once any serious condition is excluded, it is safe to use self-medica-tion. Take one tablet morning and night, for two weeks a month starting a week after the period has stopped.

• For pain on the right: PALLADIUM 6C and MUREX 6C

• For pain on the left: LACHESIS 6C

• For pain on both sides: PLATINA 6C and CIMICIFUGA 6C

Uterine fibroids

Fibroids are commonly found in women aged between 40 and 50, and often respond remarkably well to homeopathic remedies. Such treatment should only be instigated by a homeo-path.

Vaginal discharge

Vaginal discharge is normal if it remains light and clear. If this is not the case, consult your doctor for an exami-nation. There are a variety of causes of vaginal discharge. Once reassured there is no other treatment needed, take one tablet of one of the following morning and night:

• When there is a very watery discharge with itching: ALUMINA 6C.

• For a runny discharge like an egg white: BORAX 6C

• For a discharge that looks like milk curd, with itching: HELONIAS 6C

• When there is a yellow discharge, but no irritation: PULSATILLA 6C

• When there is a yellow discharge with irritation and a foul smell: KREOSO-TUM 6C

• When there is a greenish, irritating discharge that is more copious at night: MERCURIUS VIVUS 6C

Breasts

Breast pain is often due to hormonal changes during the menstrual cycle and is discussed in 'Period problems'. Chronic breast pain and cysts require a medical consultation and appropriate investigations. PHYTOLACCA is a remedy that your homeopath may recommend.

Solitary breast lumps always need full investigation to exclude cancer. It is very rare indeed for a painful lump to be cancerous.

Note: Breast swelling is common in boys at the onset of puberty. It is due to hormonal changes. They should be reassured, as the symptom will disappear in a few months.

Fever

It is always important to identify the cause of a fever, which will entail medical investigations. Homeopathy has the advantage of being able to provide risk-free treatment while that cause is being investigated.

Select the remedy that corresponds most closely to the signs and symptoms below and take one tablet three times a day:

• The high fever comes on suddenly, after exposure to dry cold weather. The skin is red and dry. The person is shivering, anxious, and restless. There is an intense thirst for cold water: ACONITE 6C

• Following exposure to the biting cold or intense sun (sunstroke), there is a high fever, with shivering. The skin is red and hot, damp with sweat particularly on the face. The person is exhausted, and may suffer from delirium. Better for cooling, aggravated by the light: BELLADONNA 6C

• The fever is slight (100.4–102.2 ° F/ 38–39 ° C). The face alternates between pallor and redness. The sweating is sometimes profuse but does not bring relief. Nosebleeds may occur. The fever often precedes upper respiratory tract infections, bronchitis, tracheitis, or an ear infection: FERRUM PHOSPHORICUM 6C

• Shivering starts prior to the fever. The mouth is very dry and there is intense thirst. The person is motionless, as every movement hurts, and drinks a lot of water. This is often seen with influenza: BRYONIA 6C

• The fever is high, with intense shivering and trembling. Shivers run down the back. The person is weak, unable to move in bed, and aches all over. The face is red and congested, and there are profuse exhausting sweats. Thirst is absent. The onset of influenza: GELSEMIUM 6C

• The onset of the fever is sudden, often with associated tonsillitis. The person is dry or sweats intermittently. The pains are sharp and burning in nature; cold improves them. There may be swelling or oedema. Heat aggravates the symptoms. The person is never thirsty: APIS MELLIFICA 6C

• Classic fever of influenza: high, with shivering when the subject is uncovered. Intense aching in all the bones, muscles, and joints. The more intense the shivering, the more profuse the sweating: EUPATORIUM PERFOLIATUM 6C

• There is a mild fever that comes and goes. The person is very sensitive, with strange feelings of hot or cold in various parts of the body. Shivering even in a hot room, aggravated by heat. Need for fresh air. There is no thirst. The onset of an infectious disease or during convalescence: PULSATILLA 6C

• There is a high fever of sudden onset, after a cold snap in the weather, a temper fit, or the emergence of baby teeth. At first the person is not thirsty, then there is profuse sweating on the head and face, with very intense thirst. The person is very restless, bad tempered, irritable, and extremely sensitive to pain and the slightest setback. In the case of a child, he or she is improved by being taken in the arms and, in cases of teething, one cheek appears redder and hotter than the other: CHAMOMILLA 6C

• Periodic fevers in weak people, often anaemic, dry at first, with shivering and no thirst. Then profuse sweating and thirst appear. The fever recurs, often on alternate days: CHINA 6C

• There is a high fever after a trauma or overexertion. Hot, red head and face,

with the rest of the body cold. The skin feels sensitive all over, as if bruised. The person is restless and cannot get comfortable. Periods of delirium alternating with periods of prostration: ARNICA 6C

• The fever follows slight exposure to cold (a mere draught) in a strong, sedentary, highly sensitive, irritable subject prone to overeating and the abuse of alcohol and coffee. The slightest feeling of cold (being uncovered) aggravates shivering. Extra clothing or heating in the room does not bring any improvement: NUX VOMICA 6C

• The fever in infectious diseases leads to restlessness, slight delirium, and profound weakness. Generalized pain and aching that make the subject continually change position: RHUS TOXICODENDRON 6C

• High feverish state following food poisoning or an infection. Great need for heat and fresh air. There is an intense thirst for small amounts of water, with a tendency to vomiting. Periods of excitability alternate with periods of collapse. All the symptoms are aggravated between midnight and 3 a.m.: ARSENICUM ALBUM 6C

In cases of serious infections, your homeopath may prescribe PYROGEN.

Warning
Do not administer antibiotics at the onset of fever as this makes diagnosis difficult.

Fidgeting

Fidgetiness can be a minor behavioural problem but it is also found in many illnesses and disease states.

• People who are always in a hurry and 'short of time' will benefit from ARGENTUM NITRICUM 6C, one tablet three to four times a day

• In cases of fidgeting with facial tics, take AGARICUS MUSCARIUS 6C, one tablet three to four times a day

• In cases of constant fidgeting with the hands, take KALI BROMATUM 6C, one tablet three to four times a day

• In cases of acute fever with fidgeting, take ACONITE 6C, one tablet every hour until an improvement is noted

Fissures

See 'Skin, hair, and nails'.

Flatulence

See 'Abdominal wind' under 'Digestive disorders'.

Folliculitis

An infection usually caused by the bacterium Staphylococcus, which develops at the root of a hair. Disinfect by alternating a mild antiseptic with a diluted solution of mother tincture CALENDULA (30 drops in a bowl of water).

Take BELLADONNA 6C, FERRUM PHOSPHORICUM 6C, and HEPAR SULPH 6C, one tablet of each three times a day.

Food cravings

See 'Cravings'.

Food intolerance

See 'Allergies'.

Fractures

See 'Traumas and burns'

Frigidity

See 'Sexual problems'.

Fungal infections

Fungal infections are very difficult to eradicate. Topical treatment, with antifungal preparations, frequently does not bring about a permanent cure.

If the infection persists, constitutional remedies prescribed by a homeopath may resolve the problem. Recurrent fungal infections are a sign that the immune system is not working at its best. See your doctor for a check-up unless the infection is very superficial, such as athlete's foot. While waiting, you can take:

• For thrush in the mouth of children:

BORAX 6C, MERCURIUS VIVUS 6C, and CANDIDA ALBICANS 6C, one tablet of each, three times a day

• For fungal infections of the nails, which have grown thicker: ANTIMONIUM CRUDUM 6C and GRAPHITES 6C, one tablet of each, three times a day

• For fungal infections of the skin and intertrigo (rash caused by a fungal infection in the skin creases): ARSENICUM IODATUM 6C, and GRAPHITES 6C, one tablet of each, three times a day

• For athlete's foot: GRAPHITES 6C and NITRIC ACID 6C, one tablet of each, three times a day

• For vaginal thrush: HELONIAS 6C and CANDIDA ALBICANS 6C, one tablet of each, three times a day

Furred tongue

See 'The Mouth'.

Gallstones

See 'Colic' and 'Diarrhoea'.

Gastritis

See 'Acidity' under 'Digestive disorders'.

German measles

See 'Childhood illnesses'.

Gingivitis

See 'Gums' under 'The Mouth'.

Glands, swelling of

Infections or wounds can lead to swelling of the neighbouring lymph glands. These are readily noticed in the neck, armpits, and groin. Certain tumours can also be associated with swollen glands. A doctor should always investigate swollen glands.

Swollen glands in the neck are common in children prone to recurrent infections of the ear, nose, and throat. Your homeopath will be able to treat them, using remedies such as HEPAR SULPH, SILICA, SULPHUR IODATUM, and THUJA. It is not advisable to use them in self-medication.

Glandular fever

This viral disease is common in adolescents. There is a very painful sore throat, swollen glands in the neck, a fever, and very intense fatigue. The doctor will make the diagnosis from a blood test.

While awaiting the results, take MERCURIS CORROSIVUS 6C and PHYTOLACCA 6C three times a day.

During the convalescence, which often lasts up to three months, take KALI PHOSPHORICUM 6C twice daily.

Glaucoma

Glaucoma is a serious eye disorder with increased pressure within the eye. Self-medication is out of the question so you must see a doctor, who will refer you to an eye specialist.

Goitre

Goitre is an increase in the size of the thyroid glands in the neck. No self-medication is possible and a doctor must be consulted.

Gout

Uric acid is deposited in the joints, which then become red, hot, and very painful. Take COLCHICUM 6C and BELLADONNA 6C, one tablet of each every hour for as long as the crisis lasts. A homeopath will prescribe a constitutional remedy.

Grazes

All grazes must be disinfected twice a day until they heal, using a solution of mother tincture of CALENDULA (30 drops in a bowl of water). This is a very effective natural disinfectant. The wounds must be cleaned thoroughly with soap and water before using CALENDULA.

Grief

See 'Depression'.

Grinding of teeth

This symptom, also known as bruxism, can be found in both children and adults and can be treated with homeopathy. Take one tablet of the suitable remedy in the morning and evening:

• In a nervous child with pinworms: CINA 6C

• In a child during teething: CHAMOMILLA 6C and PODPHYLLUM 6C

• With night terrors, in both children and adults: STRAMONIUM 6C and HYOSCYMUS 6C

• With toothache: COFFEA 6C

Gums

See 'The Mouth'.

Gynaecomastia (breast swelling in men)

This occurs during puberty in young boys and is due to hormonal changes. It is temporary and usually resolves in a few months.

Two homeopathic remedies can help: CALCAREA CARBONICA 6C and NATRUM MURIATICUM 6C taken twice daily.

Warning

In adult men it is a serious condition, requiring prompt medical attention.

Haemorrhages and bleeding

An acute haemorrhage is the flow of blood from an artery or vein. It is an emergency, sometimes requiring surgery. The bleeding must be stopped and the cause found.

Never panic. Bleeding is always dramatic but the amount of blood lost is often minimal; the main priority is to discover its source as quickly as possible. It is essential to call the doctor immediately, unless the bleeding is trivial when there is less urgency.

Anal fissure
• NITRIC ACID 6C, GRAPHITES 6C, PAEONIA 6C, and RATANHIA 6C, one tablet of each morning and night

• After the bleeding episode, or to prevent its return, take CHINA 6C, MILLEFOLIUM 6C, and FERRUM PHOSPHORICUM 6C, one tablet in the morning and evening. It is important to visit a doctor to see if further treatment is necessary

Haemorrhoids (piles)

Whatever the symptoms, combine the following remedies:

• LACHESIS 6C, MURIATIC ACID 6C, ARNICA 6C, and AESCULUS HIP-

POCASTANUM 6C, one tablet in the morning and evening, and every 15 minutes when a problem occurs. Lengthen the interval between doses once there is an improvement.

Nosebleed

• MILLEFOLIUM 6C, ARNICA 6C, and CHINA 6C, one tablet every 10 minutes when the nose is bleeding, and twice daily for two weeks afterwards.

Hair loss

See 'Skin, hair, and nails'.

Hay fever

This disease is very tiresome because of the length of time it lasts (from two to three months) and its annual recurrence, but it responds well to homeopathic remedies.

From the beginning of March, take one granule or tablet of the following remedies in the morning and evening : HISTAMINE 6C daily and MIXED POLLENS AND GRASSES 30C weekly.

Add one tablet several times a day of one of the following remedies:

• Runny nose, causing irritation of the skin of the nose and sneezing fits: ALLIUM CEPA 6C

• For red watery eyes and runny nose without skin irritation: EUPHRASIA 6C

• When the nose is running constantly,

causing a great deal of skin irritation, and there is excessive sneezing: NAPHTHALINE 6C

• For repeated sneezing and itching at the back of the throat: SABADILLA 6C

• For sneezing triggered off by draughts: NUX VOMICA 6C

Note: Constitutional homeopathic treatment can reduce the allergic tendency.

Headaches and migraines

When a headache starts, take a rest in peaceful surroundings, free of sensory stimuli (noise, light).

Recurrent headaches generally require constitutional treatment. However, it is worth trying to curb them by taking, according to the situation, one tablet of one or two remedies every 15 minutes:

• After a cold snap in the weather: ACONITE 6C and BELLADONNA 6C.

• After constipation: BRYONIA 6C

• After an emotional setback or disappointment: IGNATIA 6C and NATRUM MURIATICUM 6C

• After sunstroke: GLONOINE 6C and APIS MELLIFICA 6C

• After a hearty meal washed down with plenty of alcohol: NUX VOMICA 6C

• After great muscular exertion: ARNICA 6C and RHUS TOXICODENDRON 6C

• After intellectual effort: CALCAREA PHOSPHORICA 6C and KALI PHOSPHORICUM 6C

• Triggered by cold, damp weather: DULCAMARA 6C

• Following a minor knock on the head: NATRUM MURIATICUM 6C and NATRUM SULPHURICUM 6C

• From eye strain: RUTA 6C and ONOSMODIUM 6C

• During periods: CIMICUGA 6C

• Triggered by high altitudes: COCA 6C

• With throbbing pain aggravated by noise and light: BELLADONNA 6C

• Pain aggravated by the slightest movement or by coughing: BRYONIA 6C

• As a result of travel sickness: COCCULUS 6C

• Aggravated by coffee: NUX VOMICA 6C

• Aggravated by tea: THUJA 6C

• Aggravated by wine: NUX VOMICA 6C and ZINCUM 6C

• Aggravated by, or triggered by, a storm: PHOSPHORUS 6C and RHODODENDRON 6C

• On the right-hand side: SAN-GUINARIA 6C

• On the left-hand side: SPIGELIA 6C.

• With vomiting and eye problems: IRIS VESICOLOR 6C

• With abundant diarrhoea and cold sweats: VERATRUM ALBUM 6C

Warning
Persistent or recurrent headaches must be fully investigated.

Heartburn

See 'Digestive disorders'.

Heat stroke and sunburn

The sun that gives us life can also be dangerous. When we expose ourselves to its rays for too long there can be serious consequences: heat stroke or sunstroke. Headaches of varying intensity appear, with aching all over the body, and temperature regulation can be affected in serious cases.

Put the subject in the shade, make him or her drink, and monitor the body temperature.

• Sunstroke: APIS MELLIFICA 6C, one tablet every 15 minutes, spacing out the remedy when an improvement is noticed

• Heat stroke. Following a more intense exposure to heat, take ACONITE 6C, one tablet every 15 minutes, until sweating starts. Then change to BELLADONNA 6C, one tablet every 15 minutes, reducing the frequency when an improvement is noted

Warning
When the condition is more serious, following a prolonged exposure to the sun, with increased body temperature and restlessness with delirium, hospitalization is required.

Heel pains

See 'Osteoarthritis'.

Hepatitis

The first symptom of hepatitis is jaundice.

This symptom requires immediate medical attention and a complete check-up to make an exact diagnosis. Hepatitis can be viral, parasitic, toxic, or due to an obstruction in the gall bladder, such as a gallstone.

Once full investigations have been performed, PHOSPHORUS 6C twice daily may be beneficial. A professional homeopath may prescribe additional remedies.

Herpes (cold sores)

These outbreaks of painful blisters reappear on the lips and the nostrils, often with a mild fever. They respond well to homeopathy, providing the treatment starts early when the skin starts to itch, before the small blisters appear.

• Take APIS MELLIFICA 6C, one tablet every 15 minutes for two hours

• If the blisters appear take RHUS TOX-ICODENDRON 6C, one tablet four times a day

Warning
Herpes blisters are highly contagious!

Hiatus hernia

See 'Digestive disorders'.

Hiccups

Hiccups are caused by spasmodic contractions of the diaphragm and respond well to homeopathic remedies, both in breast-feeding babies and in adults:

• CUPRUM METALLICUM 6C, IGNATIA 6C, and HYOSCYMUS 6C, one tablet of each at every feed in babies, in adults the same remedies every two hours

High blood pressure

High blood pressure may be treated with homeopathy alongside conventional medication. Consult your homeopath.

Hip arthritis

See 'Arthritis' and 'Osteoarthritis'.

Hoarseness

See 'Laryngitis'.

Hot flushes

See 'Menopause'.

Hunger

This can be a guide to a choice of constitutional remedy.

• Greediness with constant hunger between meals: ANTIMONIUM CRUDUM

• Gnawing hunger after meals: LYCOPODIUM, PHOSPHORUS, IODUM and STAPHYSAGRIA

• Hunger at night: PHOSPHORUS, PSORINUM, CHINA, and ABIES NIGRA

• Irregular appetite, fussy about food: IGNATIA and MAGNESIA MURIATICA

• Ravenous hunger around 10 or 11 a.m.: NATRUM MURIATICUM

• Ravenous hunger around midday: SULPHUR

• Ravenous hunger around 5 p.m.: LYCOPODIUM

• Ravenous hunger during migraines: PSORINUM

• Ravenous hunger in emotional or nervous states: IGNATIA

Hyperglycaemia (high blood sugar)

See 'Diabetes'.

Hypoglycaemia (low blood sugar)

This can occur in young children and women when their reserves of sugar are insufficient. They feel faint, sweat profusely, and are shaky.

Make the child or woman drink something sweet as soon as possible. Give a tablet of LYCOPODIUM 30C as soon as this occurs, then BELLADONNA 6C and SENNA 6C, one tablet every half-hour for the next three hours.

A homeopath will prescribe remedies, such as LYCOPODIUM, NATRUM MURIATICUM, SEPIA, IGNATIA, or PHOSPHORUS, to prevent recurrence.

Impetigo

This pustular rash, which spreads on the skin of the face, is caused by infection with the bacterium Streptococcus or Staphylococcus. It is found in children who are run down.

Start the treatment as quickly as possible because impetigo is very contagious!

While waiting to see the doctor: MEZEREUM 6C, GRAPHITES 6C, and CALCAREA CARBONICA 6C, one tablet of each four times a day.

Disinfect the area with diluted CALENDULA (10 drops of mother tincture in a glass of water). Consult a homeopath for a constitutional remedy.

Impotence

See 'Sexual problems'.

Indigestion

See 'Digestive disorders'.

Influenza

Influenza is an epidemic viral disease that affects millions of people every year. It is characterized by fever, severe weakness, and generalized muscle pains that force people to stay in bed.

It is important to keep warm and drink plenty of water.

Take COLD AND FLU 30C once a week from the beginning of October to the end of February.

As soon as the first symptoms appear, choose the most appropriate remedy for the fever (See 'Fever'). Take one granule or tablet every hour, decreasing the frequency when you notice an improvement.

If the choice seems too difficult, combine the most likely remedies: GELSEMIUM 6C, EUPATORIUM PERFOLIATUM 6C, BRYONIA 6C, and RHUS TOXICODENDRON 6C.

There are no homeopathic vaccinations. Elderly people who are offered the conventional vaccine should take a dose of THUJA 30C the day before, the day of vaccination, and the following day.

Take plenty of rest at home, to avoid the risk of serious complications, such as pneumonia.

Insect bites

See 'Trauma and burns'.

Insomnia

See 'Sleep and sleep disturbances'.

Itching

Itching produces an irresistible urge to scratch. It often gives rise to skin infections. There may be an underlying disease causing the itching, so it is advisable to see your doctor.

Take DOLICHOS 6C and STAPHYSAGRIA 6C, one tablet morning and night, plus one of the following remedies:

• In cases of intense itching, take the remedies several times a day (up to once every 30 minutes):

• After an emotional setback or disappointment: IGNATIA 6C

• Burning itching improved by heat: ARSENICUM ALBUM 6C

• Burning itching improved by cold: SULPHUR 6C

• Very violent itching aggravated by scratching: MEZEREUM 6C

• Feeling of being pricked, as if by needles: URTICA URENS 6C

• Aggravated by exposure to air, particularly when undressing: RUMEX CRISPUS 6C

• Aggravated by wool: HEPAR SULPH 6C

• Aggravated by the slightest contact: RANUNCULUS BULBOSUS 6C

Warning
Itching can be the first symptom of a serious disease.

Jaundice

See 'Hepatitis'.

Joint pains

See also 'Arthritis' and 'Osteoarthritis'.

• Sciatica (lumbago) is pain along the course of the sciatic nerve, caused by

Joint pains

inflammation around the joints of the lumbar vertebrae (as with a slipped disc)

• Tendonitis is an inflammation of the tendons after unaccustomed physical activity or excessive sport

• Torticollis is a painful contraction of the neck muscles

Rest as much as possible when you experience pain. See a doctor if the symptoms do not settle quickly. An osteopath may help with sciatic pain or a stiff neck.

Sciatica

Take, according to the situation, one tablet, four times a day, of one of the following remedies:

• Pain aggravated when sitting: AMMONIUM MURIATICUM 6C

• Pain aggravated by the slightest movement: BRYONIA 6

• Pain aggravated when standing up: SULPHUR 6C

• Pain aggravated by humidity: RHUS TOXICODENDRON 6C and DULCAMARA 6C

• Pain aggravated when leaning forward and improved when leaning back: DIOSCOREA 6C

• Pain along the entire course of the sciatic nerve: HYPERICUM 6C and MAGNESIA PHOSPHORICA 6C

• Pain following injury: ARNICA 6C and RUTA 6C

• Pain aggravated at night: KALI IODATUM 6C

• Pain like electric shocks: KALMIA LATIFOLIA 6C and MAGNESIA PHOSPHORIC 6C

• Pain improved by bending the leg up to the abdomen: COLOCYNTHIS 6C

Tendonitis

Inflammation of a tendon may follow unaccustomed physical activity or excessive sport. Take RHUS TOXICODENDRON 6C and RUTA 6C, one tablet of each morning and night, until there is improvement.

Stiff neck (torticollis)

This painful contraction of the neck muscles responds well to homeopathy. Take LACHNANTHES 6C, BRYONIA 6C, and CIMICIFUGA 6C, one tablet of each three times a day, then less frequently once you notice an improvement.

Joint swelling

Fluid may collect in a joint following injury, inflammation or infection.

Consult a doctor in all cases, as X-rays and a medical examination will be required.

While waiting for a consultation, take APIS MELLIFICA 6C and BRYONIA 6C, one tablet of each every 30 minutes, decreasing the frequency when you notice an improvement.

Knee pains

See 'Arthritis' and 'Osteoarthritis'.

Knocks and blows

See 'Trauma and burns'.

Laryngitis

This is usually viral in origin and leads to pain, fever, hoarseness, and sometimes voice loss. It is common in young children.

The symptoms can be alarming in children, as the swelling may lead to breathing difficulties. Call a doctor immediately if this occurs. Whilst waiting you can try homeopathic remedies: ACONITE 6C, SPONGIA TOSTA 6C, and SAMBUCUS NIGRA 6C, one tablet of each every 15 minutes, reducing the frequency as there is improvement.

Consult a doctor if laryngitis persists or recurs frequently in an adult. This may be a sign of a serious health problem.

Leg pains

Take one tablet of each remedy morning and night:

• For heavy legs due to varicose veins: AESCULUS HIPPOCASTANUM 6C, ARNICA 6C, HAMAMELIS 6C, and FLU-ORIC ACID 6C

• For fidgety legs: ZINCUM 6C and CUPRUM METALLICUM 6C

• For muscle and joint pains: ARNICA 6C, RHUS TOXICODENDRON 6C, and CAUSTICUM 6C

Libido

See 'Sexual problems'.

Lichen planus

Lichen planus is a skin disease consisting of small red papules that itch very intensely. These lesions are usually found on the arms and wrists but they can extend all over the body. The cause of this disease is unknown. A constitutional treatment prescribed by a homeopath is required. Meanwhile, take ARSENICUM IODATUM 6C, ANACARDIUM ORIENTALE 6C, and RHUS TOXICODENDRON 6C, one tablet of each, morning and night.

Ligaments

Ligaments can be damaged after sprains or dislocations, and must be rested as advised by your doctor. Two homeopathic remedies are very effective in promoting healing: RUTA 6C and RHUS TOXICODENDRON 6C, one tablet of each three times a day for one to two weeks.

Lips

• Dry lips split vertically down the middle, aggravated by cold weather: NATRUM MURIATICUM 6C, one tablet three times a day until the lip heals

• Dry lips with cracks over a yellow base in the corner of the mouth: GRAPHITES 6C, one tablet three times a day until the lip heals

• Dry lips with cracks over a red base in the corner of the mouth: NITRIC ACID 6C, one tablet three times a day until the lip heals

Low blood pressure

Low blood pressure can have a number of causes and therefore needs to be investigated by a doctor. It is often found in states of fatigue, and can be treated by homeopathy (see 'Fatigue').

Lumbago

See 'Joint pains'.

Lump in the throat

See 'Nerves, fear, and anxiety'.

Lymphangitis

Following infection or trauma, the lymphatic vessels may become inflamed. You may feel an enlarged gland nearby.

If there is no improvement in 24 hours, see your doctor.

Take, as soon as possible: ARNICA 6C and RANA BUFO 6C, one tablet of each, four times a day. Along the painful red path of the duct, apply a compress soaked in diluted CALENDULA (10 drops of mother tincture in a glass of warm water).

Malnutrition

All weight loss must be fully investigated by your doctor. Constitutional remedies can assist in weight gain once the cause is found. The following combination can be helpful: CALCAREA PHOSPHORICA 6C, SILICA 6C, NATRUM MURIATICUM 6C, and KALI PHOSPHORICUM 6C, one tablet of each three times a day for two months, with appropriate mineral and vitamin supplements.

Measles

See 'Childhood illnesses'.

Memory disorders

Memory can diminish with age, but this can be reduced by regular mental activity. Everybody should make the effort to learn something new every day throughout his or her life. Constitutional remedies can help to maintain intellectual function.

Add one tablet of the following remedies twice a day:

• For problems with the memory due to intellectual overexertion: ANACARDIUM ORIENTALE 6C and KALI PHOSPHORICUM 6C

• For memory loss due to ageing: BARYTA CARBONICA 6C and THUJA 6C

Meningitis

Meningitis is a life-threatening inflammation of the coverings of the brain. It presents with headache, neck stiffness, fever, rash, drowsiness, and vomiting.

This is a medical emergency that requires hospital treatment.

If it is bacterial meningitis it must be treated with antibiotics.

If it is viral meningitis, there is no specific medical treatment.

Menopause

The menopause occurs in women when the ovaries stop producing eggs. Hot flushes may occur in association with the hormonal changes. In view of the problems with hormone replacement therapy (HRT), it is worth trying homeopathic remedies, which can give remarkable results.

As soon as the periods start to be irregular, take: FOLLICULINUM 30C once a week and LACHESIS 6C once a day,

This treatment produces excellent results in most women, but it can be improved by consulting your homeopath for a constitutional remedy.

As regards the menopausal symptoms:

Hot flushes
• On the face with profuse sweating: BELLADONNA 6C, one tablet morning and evening

• Throbbing in the neck and limbs: GLONOINE 6C, one tablet morning and evening

• Triggered by emotions, with a lump in the throat: IGNATIA 6C, one tablet morning and evening

• With migraine above the right eye and burning cheeks: SANGUINARIA 6C, one tablet morning and evening

• With feelings of anxiety and palpitations: AMYL NITROSUM 6C, one tablet morning and evening

Depression

SEPIA 6C, STAPHYSAGRIA 6C, and THUJA 6C, one tablet of each, in the morning and evening, during the difficult spell. Please consult a doctor if the depression is severe or does not respond quickly to treatment.

Osteoporosis

CALCAREA PHOSPHORICA 6C and SYMPHYTUM 6C, one tablet of each, morning and evening, every other month during the menopause may help prevent osteoporosis. Ensure that you have a good source of calcium, such as cheese or milk. Physical exercise (especially walking) also seems to be beneficial.

Menstruation

See 'Period problems'.

Migraines

See 'Headaches and migraines'.

Modalities

Modalities are the factors which modify the symptom picture. Each remedy has a unique set of modalities, which the homeopath uses as a guide to finding an appropriate remedy. Certain conditions improve the condition and others aggravate it.

For example, hot drinks improve the complaints of a LYCOPODIUM state, whereas those of a BRYONIA state are improved by cold drinks. Hot baths aggravate SULPHUR and LACHESIS, whilst cold baths aggravate ANTIMONIUM CRUDUM.

These modalities are listed in the descriptions of the remedies in Part 3.

Molluscum contagiosum

This viral infection results in multiple soft, almost spherical warts. It is fre-quently seen in children and is highly contagious. The warts are most often found on the face, the trunk, and the anal and genital areas.

Take THUJA 6C once a week, and DUL-CAMARA 6C with NITRIC ACID 6C, one tablet of each three times a day, for two to three months. Homeopathic treatment may prevent recurrence.

Moon

The various phases of the moon influence our behaviour. Certain remedy types show the influence of the moon. Thus:

• Aggravation when there is a full moon: SULPHUR, PHOSPHORUS, NATRUM MURIATICUM, CALCAREA CARBONICA, CINA, SEPIA, and SILICA

• Aggravation when there is a new moon: KALI BROMATUM, STAPHYSAGRIA, and CAUSTICUM

• Aggravation when there is a waning moon: THUJA, DULCAMARA, and IODUM

• Aggravation when there is a waxing moon: THUJA, STAPHYSAGRIA, ALUMINA, ARSENICUM ALBUM, and CLEMATIS ERECTA

• Aggravation by exposure to moonlight: ANTIMONIUM CRUDUM, ARGENTUM NITRICUM, and THUJA

Mountain sickness

See 'Altitude sickness'.

The mouth

The most common disorders found in the mouth are ulcers, a 'furred' tongue, bad breath, excessive salivation, and bleeding gums.

The mouth is in constant contact with the outside world and thus a huge variety of germs. Despite this, it is very resistant and has remarkable healing powers. Improved oral hygiene is often enough to return to a state of health.

Ulcers

Ulcers occurring inside the mouth, cheeks, and tongue are small and superficial, but very painful. They tend to recur.

As soon as the first symptoms appear, take the following combination: MERCURIUS CORROSIVUS 6C, SULPHURIC ACID 6C, BORAX 6C, and SECALE CORNUTUM 6C, one tablet of each every hour, then space the remedies as the symptoms improve. Rinse the mouth out three times a day with diluted CALENDULA (10 drops of mother tincture in a glass of warm water).

Gums

The gums can become inflamed and bleed; this is known as gingivitis. Take the following remedies: MERCURIUS VIVUS 6C and PHOSPHORUS 6C, one tablet every hour, decreasing the frequency when you notice an improve-

ment. If there is danger of abscess formation, add HEPAR SULPH 6C, one tablet morning and evening.

Bad breath

First ensure that oral hygiene is adequate and the diet is balanced. Then take: MERCURIUS VIVUS 6C, one tablet in the morning and evening for several weeks.

Tongue

This reflects the state of the digestive system and oral hygiene. Take one tablet of the chosen remedies, morning and evening:

• For a tongue with a whitish coat: ANTIMONIUM CRUDUM 6C and KALI PHOSPHORICUM 6C

• For a tongue with a yellowish coat: NUX VOMICA 6C, CHELEDONIUM 6C, and PULSATILLA 6C

• For 'geographical' tongue (some areas furred and others with no coat): NATRUM MURIATICUM and TARAXACUM 6C

• For a very heavily furred tongue, with the edges revealing the imprint of the teeth: MERCURIUS VIVUS 6C

A persistently furred tongue is often a sign of digestive problems and requires a consultation with a homeopath.

Thrush

A mouth infection caused by the fungus Candida albicans, it is often found fol-

Homeopathy encyclopedia

lowing a course of antibiotics which destroy the normal bacteria, thus undermining the natural protection against the fungus.

Take one tablet, four times a day, for two weeks, of CANDIDA ALBICANS 6C and MERCURIUS VIVUS 6C.

Excessive salivation

This symptom can have a number of causes, including psychological ones. It is therefore necessary to consult a homeopath so that he or she can choose the constitutional remedies. While waiting for the consultation, take MERCURIUS VIVUS 6C, one tablet morning and evening.

Movement

The effect of movement on the symptoms applies to many conditions, especially joint pains:

• Joint pains improved by movement, after a short warm-up: RHUS TOXICODENDRON 6C, one tablet three times a day

• Joint pains aggravated by the slightest movement: BRYONIA 6C, one tablet three times a day

Mumps

See 'Childhood illnesses'.

Muscle cramps

These are often due to insufficient warm-up before exercise. Take ARNICA 6C, MAGNESIA PHOSPHORICA 6C, and CUPRUM METALLICUM 6C, one tablet every 15 minutes when the problem occurs and one tablet morning and evening until there is improvement.

Music

Certain remedy types are better for music. These include: TARENTULA HISPANICA, IGNATIA, PULSATILLA (soft music), NATRUM MURIATICUM, AURUM METALLICUM, THUJA, PHOSPHORUS, GRAPHITES, LYCOPODIUM, CAUSTICUM, TUBERCULINUM RESIDUUM, and BUFO RANA.

Nails

See 'Skin, hair, and nails'.

Nappy rash

Nappy rash often occurs during teething. Wash the baby with a gentle soap and dry the skin thoroughly. Give the baby CHAMOMILLA 6C and ARSENICUM ALBUM 6C, one tablet of each morning and evening.

If blistering of the skin occurs, add one tablet of CROTON TIGLIUM 6C.

Neck pains

See 'Osteoarthritis'.

Nerves, fear, and anxiety

Nerves, fear, and anxiety are caused by a failure to come to terms with the unknown and the future, and always have repercussions on the physical body.

Controlling your breathing is essential if you are to keep calm.

Nervous states

Generalized nervous conditions
An in-depth consultation with a professional homoeopath is necessary to treat non-specific fears and anxiety.

While waiting for this consultation, take a combination of the remedies, proven by experience to be highly effective. Take one tablet of each, morning and night:

• For children: LACHESIS 6C, CHAMOMILLA 6C, and STRAMONIUM 6C

• For men: NUX VOMICA 6C and COLOCYNTHIS 6C

• For women: IGNATIA 6C and CIMICIFUGA 6C

Specific nervous states
Anticipation of a forthcoming event makes the person hot and bothered, too anxious to complete the task at hand: ARGENUM NITRICUM 6C, one tablet morning and night and every 15 minutes during the episode.

A sudden attack of nerves causes the person to freeze, unable to think clearly: GELSEMIUM 6C one tablet in the morning and night and every 15 minutes during the episode.

Examinations
One month before the exams, take this combination each week:

• one tablet of SILICA 6C each morning, and one tablet of each of the following, morning and night:

• IGNATIA 6C, GELSEMIUM 6C, and

• KALI PHOSPHORICUM 6C

Before and during the exams, if necessary take:

• one tablet of GELSEMIUM 6C and ARGENTUM NITRICUM 6C, as many times as needed to calm the nerves.

Fear

Fear can be difficult to control. Take, according to the situation, one tablet a day (or more often if necessary) of the chosen remedies:

• Fear of a crowd: ARGENTUM NITRICUM 6C and ACONITE 6C

• Fear of sickness: PHOSPHORUS 6C

• Fear of death: ACONITE 6C and ARSENICUM ALBUM 6C

• Fear of thunder storms: PHOSPHORUS 6C and RHODODENDRON 6C

• Fear of the dark: STRAMONIUM 6C and PHOSPHORUS 6C

Homeopathy encyclopedia

• Fear of animals: HYOSCYMUS 6C and STRAMONIUM 6C

• Fear of burglars: NATRUM MURI-ATICUM 6C and ARSENICUM ALBUM 6C

• Claustrophobia: ARGENTUM NITRICUM 6C

Anxiety

The physical effects of anxiety (crushing pains, palpitations, muscular spasms and lumps in the throat etc.) can make it feel unbearable at times. There are a large number of situations where anxiety may occur. A constitutional remedy is often required. The remedies suggested below are useful for the most common situations:

• Anxiety about something that is yet to happen, with a tendency to excessive haste: ARGENTUM NITRICUM 6C, one tablet every 15 minutes in the preceding two hours

• Anxiety during a fever with fear of dying, during episodes of palpitation or after a severe fright: ACONITE 6C, one tablet every hour, reducing the frequency as there is improvement

• Anxiety when alone, with restlessness alternating with depression, worse at night: ARSENICUM ALBUM 6C, one tablet every hour, reducing the frequency, as there is improvement

• Anxiety following an emotional setback, a sad event, or being told something hurtful. The feelings are kept in

and there is a heavy feeling in the chest: take IGNATIA 6C with STAPHY-SAGRIA 6C, one tablet of each every hour, reducing the frequency as there is improvement

Warning

Some cases of anxiety or uncontrollable fear can require psychotherapy.

Neuralgia

This exceptionally painful condition, where pain shoots along the length of a nerve, often responds very well to homeopathic remedies. Take, according to the situation, one tablet of the chosen remedies morning or night and every 15 minutes during an acute attack:

Facial neuralgia

• In all cases ACONITE 6C and BEL-LADONNA 6C. If the pain is on the right, add MAGNESIA PHOSPHORICA 6C. If the pain is on the left, add CEDRON 6C and SPIGELIA 6C.

Intercostal neuralgia (neuralgia of the chest wall)

• In all cases: HYPERICUM. If movement makes the pain worse, add BRY-ONIA 6C. If movement improves the pain add RHUS TOXICODENDRON 6C and RHODODENDRON 6C.

Specific modalities:

• The pain is triggered by humidity: DULCAMARA 6C

• The pain is triggered by dry, biting cold: ACONITE 6C

• The pain is very violent, appearing in a flash: KALMIA LATIFOLIA 6C and MAGNESIA PHOSPHORICA 6C

Nightmares

HYOSCYMUS 6C and STRAMONIUM 6C, one tablet of each before the evening meal. If the nightmares are frequent, they must always be combined with a constitutional remedy.

Nosebleed

See 'Haemorrhages and bleeding'.

Obesity

Obesity cannot be treated through self-medication. A change in lifestyle and diet combined with increased physical exercise is always needed to lose weight.

Homeopathic remedies act as regulators of the metabolism and therefore can very useful. A homeopath will select constitutional remedies. Patience is required; you will not lose the 45 pounds you have accumulated over 10 years in 3 months!

Warning

Certain dubious 'slimming clinics' use stimulants, diuretics, and thyroid extracts to assist with weight loss. This is extremely dangerous and cannot be too vigorously denounced!

See also 'Digestive disorders'.

Osteoarthritis

Osteoarthritis is a degenerative condition of the joints and cartilage causing stiffness, swelling, and pain.

Try to avoid anti-inflammatory drugs as these mask the symptoms, without treating the cause.

For painful attacks of osteoarthritis, take one tablet of the following remedies every hour, depending on the location of the pain, reducing the frequency when an improvement is noted:

• For the neck: FERRUM PHOSPHORICUM 6C

• For the back, between the shoulder blades: CIMICIFUGA 6C

• For the lumbar vertebrae (lower back): KALI CARBONICUM 6C

• For a bony protuberance, called a 'calcaneal spur', under the heel: HECLA LAVA 6C, one tablet morning and night

• For the base of the thumb: ACTEA SPICATA 6C

Add according to the situation:

• Pain triggered by wet weather: DULCAMARA 6C

• Pain triggered by a storm or low

Osteoarthritis

atmospheric pressure: RHODODEN-DRON 6C

• Pain triggered by an emotional set-back or anger: NUX VOMICA 6C

• For joint swelling, add APIS MELLI-FICA 6C, KALI IODATUM 6C, and BRY-ONIA 6C

A doctor should monitor your progress. A constitutional remedy and nutritional supplements are required.

Osteoporosis

See 'Osteoporosis' under 'Menopause'.

Ovarian pains

See 'Female reproductive system'.

Overeating

Certain remedies may help diminish cravings for particular food items. Take one tablet of 6C before eating:

• Overeating in general: ANTIMONIUM CRUDUM and NUX VOMICA
• Alcohol: NUX VOMICA
• Beer: KALI BICHROMICUM
• Butter and fat: PULSATILLA and CARBO VEGETABILIS
• Cakes: CARBO VEGETABILIS
• Coffee: COFFEA
• Eggs: SULPHUR
• Fish and seafood: URTICA URENS
• Fizzy drinks: KALI CARBONICUM
• Fruit: CHINA

• Meat: ALLIUM SATIVUM
• Milk: MAGNESIA CARBONICA
• Onion: THUJA
• Raw vegetables: LYCOPODIUM, BERBERIS, and BRYONIA
• Salt: NATRUM MURIATICUM
• Spices: NUX VOMICA and SEPIA
• Sugar: ARGENTUM NITRICUM
• Wine: ZINCUM

See also 'Cravings'.

Palpitations

Palpitations are not always a sign of heart disease and may be due to emotional problems, which respond well to homeopathy.

Do not panic when you have an attack of palpitations; see your doctor, who will decide whether you need to consult a heart specialist. In the meantime, look at ways of reducing stress in your life.

Start taking the remedies below as soon as possible. Take one tablet of the chosen remedies every 15 minutes during an attack, and each morning and night:

• After a fright: GELSEMIUM 6C

• After violent emotions: IGNATIA 6C, MOSCHUS 6C, and AMBRA GRISEA 6C

• After too much tobacco or coffee: NUX VOMICA 6C and IGNATIA 6C

• After a big meal: LYCOPODIUM 6C and NUX VOMICA 6C

- During the menopause: LACHESIS 6C

- With anxiety and restlessness: ACONITE 6C

- Painful, with headache: SPIGELIA 6C

Parasites

See 'Worms'.

Period problems

These problems can be helped considerably by homoeopathy. If they are severe or persist, you must see a gynaecologist.

Period pains often seem to occur at night, particularly on a Sunday, so have the remedies to hand. A covered hot-water bottle placed on the stomach is often very soothing.

With all period problems take FOLLICULINUM 6C daily in the two weeks prior to your period. Add one tablet of the chosen remedies, morning and night.

Absent periods
Pregnancy must be excluded first of all. If you are not pregnant, consult your homeopath.

While waiting you can try the following remedies, according to the probable cause of the missed period:

- After getting cold and wet, or a cold bath: DULCAMARA 6C and ANTIMONIUM CRUDUM 6C

- In a shy young woman suffering with problems of the circulation: PULSATILLA 6C

- After great fatigue: MANGANUM 6C

- After a great fright: GELSEMIUM 6C and ARNICA 6C

- After an explosion of anger: CHAMOMILLA 6C

Pre-menstrual problems
- For violent stomach cramps, improved by bending over: MAGNESIA PHOSPHORICA 6C

- For headaches and dizziness before irregular, heavy periods with black blood: CYCLAMEN 6C

- For sore, lumpy breasts: PHYTOLACCA 6C

- For problems which ease immediately the period starts: LACHESIS 6C

- For painful swelling of the breasts before periods, improving during the period: LAC CANINUM 6C

Period pains
- For violent cramps, improved by bending over: COLOCYNTHIS 6C

- For light periods with lots of cramping pain: CAULOPHYLLUM 6C

- For violent cramps improved by standing very straight or leaning back: DIOSCOREA VILLOSA 6C

Period problems

Pain in the back and lower stomach
• For very painful periods with large amounts of red blood: SABINA 6C

• When the blood is dark, almost black: SECALE CORNUTUM 6C

• For pain that varies according to the intensity of the flow of blood: CIMICUGA 6C

• For intense cramps, with cold sweats and feeling icy cold: VERATRUM ALBUM 6C

• For short-lived cramps in periods that come late and are over within a few hours: VIBURNUM OPULUS 6C

• For heavy periods where the flow increases with movement: TRILIUM PENDULUM 6C

Pityriasis versicolor

A fungus causes this skin disease. Take ARSENICUM ALBUM 6C, ARSENICUM IODATUM 6C, and SEPIA 6C, one tablet of each morning and night for a month.

Pregnancy

Minor complaints may be experienced during pregnancy, which can be treated with homoeopathy. Homoeopathy is quite safe for mother and baby, but seek professional advice, as the potency needs to be adjusted in pregnancy. Your homoeopath may suggest some of the remedies listed below:

• Constipation: SEPIA and COLLINSONIA

• Contractions in the last months: CAULOPHYLLUM

• Depression during pregnancy: SEPIA

• Fear of giving birth: GELSEMIUM and CIMICIFUGA

• Haemorrhoids: COLLINSONIA, AESCULUS HIPPOCASTANUS, and ARNICA

• Hiccups: CUPRUM METALLICUM

• Excessive salivation: MERCURIUS VIVUS

• Backache: KALI CARBONICUM and SEPIA

• Nausea: IGNATIA and IPECAC

• Preparation for labour: CAULOPHYLLUM

• Varicose veins: BELLIS PERENNIS, AESCULUS HIPPOCASTANUM, and HAMAMELIS

• Vomiting: SEPIA and IGNATIA

Warning
Avoid all allopathic drugs during pregnancy, unless prescribed by your doctor, as most of them pass through the placenta.

Prolapse

The uterus and bladder may prolapse

due to a weakness in the supporting ligaments and muscles.

In most cases surgery will be required, so a medical examination is essential.

Homeopathy can help to strengthen the supporting tissues. Take SEPIA 6C and CALCAREA FLUORICA 6C, one tablet of each twice a day.

Prostate problems

The prostate gland increases in size with age, and may cause problems with the flow of urine. Homeopathy may help to delay an operation. Take THUJA 6C once a day, with SABAL SERRULATA 6C and CONIUM MACULATA 6C twice daily.

Psoriasis

See 'Skin, hair, and nails'.

Puberty and juvenile acne

The age at which sexual maturity occurs varies from individual to individual.

Every child reaches puberty at the appointed time and it is not advisable to intervene with aggressive medicines during this period. Hormonal treatments that could affect this natural process are not recommended unless prescribed by a specialist.

Puberty is often accompanied by acne. This is caused by the hormonal changes, leading to increased activity in the oil-producing glands of the skin. Infection may occur.

Puberty

Homeopathic remedies can be used to give this natural process a nudge in the right direction. In all cases, give PULSATILLA 6C, one tablet morning and night, for three to six months. Add, according to the situation:

• For a fearful and introverted adolescent, often tall and lanky: NATRUM MURIATICUM 6C daily for three to six months

• When the adolescent is worn out by the growth spurts: CALCAREA PHOSPHORICA 6C and SYMPHYTUM 6C, one tablet twice a day

• For a whining adolescent, intelligent but lacking in self-confidence: LYCOPODIUM 6C daily for three to six months

• For an emotionally unstable adolescent with nervous tics: AGARICUS MUSCARIUS daily for three to six months

Acne

• For greasy skin and blackheads, take SELENIUM 6C

• For infected painful spots add EUGENIS JAMBOSA 6C twice a day

• If the spots burn, itch, and are clus-

Homeopathy encyclopedia

tered on the face, chest, and shoulders, add KALI BROMATUM 6C twice a day

• If the spots are found in places directly over bone (the forehead, nose, or the base of the spine) take two other remedies simultaneously: LEDUM PALUSTRE 6C and CALCAREA PICRICA 6C

Two remedies are helpful for the scars of acne:

• ANTIMONIUM CRUDUM 6C, one tablet twice a day, for small, well-defined scars looking like purplish-red craters

• GRAPHITES 6C, one tablet twice a day, for unsightly, blistered scars

In all cases, use diluted CALENDULA (10 drops of mother tincture in a glass of water) as a facial wash. A constitutional remedy will enhance these treatments.

Rashes

See 'Skin, hair, and nails'.

Raynaud's syndrome

Spasms in small blood vessels make the fingers swell, turn white and then blue in the cold. On coming into the warmth, the fingers turn purplish-red. This condition is more common in women and is very painful. The cause of this disease is unknown and it is not easy to cure.

A constitutional remedy is needed. While you are waiting to see a homeopath you can take SECALE CORNUTUM 6C, TABACUM 6C, and NUX VOMICA 6C, one tablet of each three times a day.

Ringing in the ears (tinnitus)

Tinnitus is more noticeable when it is quiet, and is difficult to treat. Take CHINA SULPHURICUM 6C and GLONOINE 6C, one tablet morning and night.

If the tinnitus starts suddenly, consult a doctor at once for investigation.

Rheumatism

See 'Arthritis' and 'Osteoarthritis'.

Rosacea

See 'Skin, hair, and nails'.

Scarlet fever

See 'Childhood illnesses'.

Scars

See 'Trauma and burns'.

Sciatica and lumbar sciatica

See 'Joint pains'.

Sea

People react very differently to the sea, and this is of great interest to the homeopath. It assists in remedy selection. Thus:

• Worse by the sea: NATRUM MURIATICUM, LUETICUM, ARSENICUM ALBUM, KALI IODATUM, MAGNESIA MURIATICA, NATRUM SULPHURICUM, and SEPIA

• Worse for swimming in the sea: ARSENICUM ALBUM, RHUS TOXICODENDRON, SEPIA, and MAGNESIA MURIATICA

• Better for the sea air: MEDORRHINUM and BROMIUM

Seborrhoea

See 'Skin, hair, and nails'.

Sensitivity to cold

This is a sign suggestive of a weakened immune system. It is sometimes a sign of impending illness. It is therefore wise to consult a homeopath. Meanwhile, take SILICA 6C and DULCAMARA 6C, one tablet of each morning and night.

DENDRON, SEPIA, and MAGNESIA MURIATICA

• Better for the sea air: MEDORRHINUM and BROMIUM

Sexual problems

An alteration in sexual activity is only cause for concern if it disturbs the individual in any way. In this cases counselling may be very beneficial. Reducing one's stress levels and getting adequate rest are beneficial in every respect.

In men

Decreased libido and impotence
Take one tablet of the chosen remedies morning and night:

• For difficulty in achieving erections: CONIUM MACULATA 6C

• For impotence with a high libido, after previous sexual excesses: CALADIUM 6C

• For a drop in sexual activity with absence of desire: GRAPHITES 6C

• For feeble erections and weakness after intercourse: SELENIUM 6C

• For sexual problems due to anxiety: GELSEMIUM 6C and ARGENTUM NITRICUM 6C

• For sexual problems due to loss of self-confidence: LYCOPODIUM 6C

Sexual excitement
• For violent, prolonged, and painful erections: PICRIC ACID 6C and CANTHARIS 6C. If this symptom persists, consult a doctor

• For very violent desire with the need to seduce: PHOSPHORUS 6C

Homeopathy encyclopedia

Increased sexual excitement
• For hypersensitivity of sexual organs: PLATINA 6C

• For very strong sexual excitement: LILIUM TIGRINUM 6C and MUREX 6C

• With erotic dreams: ORIGANUM 6C

• After rejection or dissatisfaction: STAPHYSAGRIA 6C

Decreased sexual desire
In all cases: ONOSMODIUM 6C, GELSEMIUM 6C, and IGNATIA 6C, one tablet of each morning and night and before intercourse

Add one tablet of the chosen remedy, according to the situation:

• For pain during sexual intercourse in a depressed woman: SEPIA 6C

• For the total absence of desire: GRAPHITES 6C

Warning
Do not take any 'miracle cures' or 'aphrodisiacs'; if they are not dangerous, they will certainly be useless.

Shingles

See 'Skin, hair, and nails'.

Shooting pains

This specific pattern of pain is impor-

tant in that it can be a guide to certain remedies.

If it occurs with the sensation of a splinter anywhere in the body, NITRIC ACID is indicated. If it feels as though a splinter is lodged in the throat ARGENTUM NITRICUM is required, and if the feeling is deep in the larynx, HEPAR SULPH is needed.

Sinusitis

The frontal and maxillary sinuses are bony cavities in the face that can become inflamed, usually as a result of an infection. Sinusitis, which often becomes chronic, is often a consequence of an upper respiratory tract infection, which also must be treated.

Start treatment promptly as the pain can be severe. The accumulation of secretions leads to pressure within the sinus.

As soon as pain or discharge appears, take one tablet of the chosen remedy four times a day, according to the situation:

• Sticky, thick, greenish-yellow catarrh, difficult to blow out, with a blocked nose and sneezing when outdoors: KALI BICHROMICUM 6C

• Thick, yellow catarrh with a blocked nose and post-nasal catarrh: HYDRASTIS 6C

• Greenish-yellow catarrh streaked with

blood, worse at night: MERCURIUS VIVUS 6C

• Abundant watery, irritating discharge: KALI IODATUM 6C

• Yellowish catarrh with burning pains in the sinuses: MEZERIUM 6C

• At the same time, take in addition one tablet of HEPAR SULPH 6C twice a day

If the sinusitis is recurrent, consult a doctor, who may suggest an X-ray to evaluate the state of the sinuses, and start constitutional treatment after seeing a homeopath.

Skin, hair, and nails

The skin and the epidermis reflect one's general state of health so homeopathy is particularly appropriate.

Avoid steroid creams as much as possible as they only relieve the symptoms without treating the cause of the skin problem.

Calluses

These thickened areas of skin are often found in areas subject to friction, particularly on the feet and hands. Take ANTIMONIUM CRUDUM 6C and LYCOPODIUM 6C, one tablet of each, twice a day for several weeks.

Dry skin

Dry skin can be itchy or flake off. It is more common in winter. A constitu-

tional remedy prescribed by a homeopath is required.

Meanwhile, take one tablet of ALUMINA 6C, ARSENICUM ALBUM 6C, and BERBERIS VULGARIS 6C twice a day for one month.

Chapped skin

Fissures or splits in the skin appear after exposure to cold or in association with eczema. Take one tablet of AGARICUS MUSCARIUS 6C and PETROLEUM 6C twice a day for one month. If the skin bleeds, add NITRIC ACID 6C at the same dose.

Eczema

Eczema is a chronic condition with acute flare-ups. Many homeopathic remedies may be used to heal the skin.

Take the chosen remedies twice a day:

• For dry eczema: ARSENICUM ALBUM 6C and ARSENICUM IODATUM 6C

• For eczema with blisters: RHUS TOXICODENDRON 6C and CANTHARIS 6C

• For scabby, oozing eczema: GRAPHITES 6C and MEZERIUM 6C

• For cracked eczema with bleeding: NITRIC ACID 6C and PETROLEUM 6C

• For very hard, cracked eczema with no bleeding: LYCOPODIUM 6C and ANTIMONIUM CRUDUM 6C

• For eczema aggravated by water or heat, improved by cold: SULPHUR 6C

Homeopathy encyclopedia

• For eczema aggravated by sun and the seaside: NATRUM MURIATICUM 6C

• For eczema worse in winter: PETROLEUM 6C

• For eczema after a vaccination: THUJA 6C and MEZERIUM 6C

If the eczema becomes infected, wash the area with diluted CALENDULA (10) drops in a bowl of water). If there is no rapid improvement, see your doctor.

Flaking skin

If the skin flakes excessively, this can be a sign of poor general health. You should consult your homeopath. The pattern of the flaking is suggestive of certain remedies.

• Fine flaking, with the shed skin resembling flour: ARSENICUM ALBUM

• Strips of skin shed, revealing red patches of skin: NATRUM SULPHURICUM

• Scaling of the skin with scabs forming: BERBERIS

Hair loss

It is difficult to prevent male baldness, as there is a genetic basis. We all know completely bald families! However, constitutional treatment prescribed by a homeopath can often slow down the progress of baldness.

When hair falls out suddenly, in clumps, due to fungal infections, a doctor must always be consulted.

The main constitutional remedies
GRAPHITES, SEPIA, THUJA, SULPHUR, NATRUM MURIATICUM and SILICA.

The complementary remedies
THALLIUM, SELENIUM, ZINCUM, PHOSPHORIC ACID and PLUMBUM.

Nails

The appearance of the nails is often linked to that of the hair. These 'dead' parts of our body are faithful reflections of our general state of health. Changes in their growth or appearance do not escape the attention of patients, who often point them out to a homeopath. The latter will use these signs to choose the appropriate remedies.

It is often possible to start to improve the situation through self-medication. Take one tablet of the chosen remedies each morning and night, according to the state of your nails:

• Thick nails that break and barely grow any more: ANTIMONIUM CRUDUM 6C and GRAPHITES 6C

• Soft nails that break easily, with vertical cracks: THUJA 6C

• Nails that break easily, with white spots: SILICA 6C

Psoriasis

The cause of this chronic skin disease is still unknown. There is no definitive cure, but constitutional remedies prescribed by a homeopath can bring some improvement.

Looking after yourself

Try the combination: ARSENICUM ALBUM 6C, ARSENICUM IODATUM 6C, and SEPIA, one tablet of each morning and night for three months. Add, according to the symptoms:

• If the skin is very thick: GRAPHITES 6C

• When it is worse in winter: PETRO-LEUM 6C

• For the scalp: CALCAREA CARBON-ICA 6C

Rosacea

Rosacea is a skin disease characterised by dilated and congested small blood vessels on the face. The cause is unknown, but its progress can be halted by homeopathy. Try CARBO ANIMALIS 6C, SANGUINARIA 6C, and ARNICA 6C one tablet of each twice a day.

Seborrhoea and seborrhoeic dermatitis

The oil-producing glands, the seba-ceous glands, produce excessive secre-tions in this condition, particularly on the face and scalp.

Take one tablet of the chosen remedy morning and night on alternate days:

• Very greasy skin, with acne on the face and a tendency to eczema in folds of skin and on the scalp: NATRUM MURI-ATICUM 6C

• Greasy skin with sweaty scalp and hair falling out: SELENIUM 6C

• Greasy skin and flatulence: RAPH-ANUS 6C

• Greasy skin in an overweight person with warts: THUJA 6C

• Greasy skin in a constipated person: BRYONIA 6C

Shingles

This viral disease, caused by the chicken pox virus is characterized by blisters along the course of a nerve.

As soon as the first symptoms appear, immediately take: a dose of STAPHY-LOCOCCINUM 30C followed by SUL-PHUR 6C one dose six hours later. Then, start RHUS TOXICODENDRON 6C, CANTHARIS 6C, and ARSENICUM ALBUM 6C, one tablet of each every two hours, decreasing the frequency when you notice an improvement.

If the blisters turn bluish purple, or if they contain a thick, yellowish liquid, take MEZERIUM 6C and RANUNCULUS BULBOSUS 6C, one tablet of each every two hours, decreasing the frequency when you notice an improvement.

Pain that persists for several months after the rash has healed responds well to homeopathic remedies: HYPER-ICUM 6C, MAGNESIA PHOSPHORICA 6C, and CAUSTICUM 6C, one tablet of each, morning and night. If this does not settle the pain, consult a homeo-path, who will prescribe a constitu-tional treatment.

Homeopathy encyclopedia

Skin rashes

A skin rash may denote an underlying health problem, so it is important to consult your homeopath.

Meanwhile, take one tablet morning and night of the following remedies, according to the situation:

• For redness of the skin: APIS MELLI-FICA 6C and BELLADONNA 6C

• For blisters: RHUS TOXICODEN-DRON 6C and CANTHARIS 6C

• For weeping skin rashes: GRAPHITES 6C and MEZERIUM 6C

• For scaly skin rashes: ARSENICUM ALBUM 6C and ARSENICUM IODATUM 6C

• For cracked skin: NITRIC ACID 6C and PETROLEUM 6C

Sun, effects on the skin

Excessive exposure to the sun is detrimental to the skin.

Some people become sensitized to certain allergens following exposure to the sun. A red rash develops as a result of contact with the allergen, such as grass pollen or perfume. Take URTICA URENS 6C, RHUS TOXICODENDRON 6C and CANTHARIS 6C, one tablet of each three times a day, if this occurs.

Urticaria

Red weals appear on the skin as a result of an allergy. Homeopathy can be very helpful.

Take HISTAMINE 6C and URTICA URENS 6C, one tablet of each every 15 minutes. Add, according to the situation:

• For urticaria caused by water: DULCA-MARA 6C

• For burning pains improved by hot applications: ARSENICUM ALBUM 6C

Warts

These small contagious lesions are viral in origin. Homeopathy will act to improve the body's defences against viruses.

In all cases take THUJA 6C, one tablet daily. Add one tablet of the chosen remedy in the morning and evening, according to the situation:

• For hard, horny, and painful warts, on any part of the body: ANTIMONIUM CRUDUM 6C

• For wide, smooth warts, often on the back of the hand or the face: DULCA-MARA 6C

• For painful, wide, flat, cracked warts that bleed easily, often on the back of the hand: NITRIC ACID 6C

• For wide, notched warts, attached to the skin by a small base, bleeding easily, sometimes on the edge of the nails: CAUSTICUM 6C

• For warts in the anal and genital regions: see your doctor

Looking after yourself

Sleep and sleep disturbances

A healthy diet, regular physical exercise such as walking, and a reduced workload are often necessary to bring back a normal sleep pattern.

Sleepiness

Sleepiness after a meal is common after the age of 40. Take one tablet of the chosen remedy before each meal:

• Sleepiness after a meal, improved by a short nap, in a very active and irritable person: NUX VOMICA 6C

• Sleepiness after a meal, aggravated by a short nap: LYCOPODIUM 6C.

• Sleepiness at several times during the day: OPIUM 6C

• Sleepiness after a meal, which causes stomach swelling, in a person prone to depression: NUX MOSCATA 6C

Sleep apnoea

This new syndrome has been widely studied in the last ten years. Some overweight people over 40, who snore, have episodes when breathing stops while they are asleep. They wake up with headaches.

The causes of this condition are unknown. It, undoubtedly, must affect the oxygen supply to certain vital organs. Weight loss and avoiding stimulants such as alcohol, tobacco, and coffee can improve the situation.

Certain homeopathic remedies may help. Try NUX VOMICA 6C, CALCAREA CARBONICA 6C, and OPIUM 6C nightly.

Sleep walking

The person gets up and wanders around, sometimes performing complex tasks, and then goes back to bed. The next day he or she has no memory of the night's events.

This type of behaviour is found in subjects of the following constitutional types: KALI BROMATUM and STRAMONIUM.

Insomnia of recent onset

This is often simply a symptom related to overwork, fatigue, and personal or professional worries. A review of your lifestyle is therefore in order, as well as an appointment with a homeopath to find a constitutional remedy.

• Take 10 drops of PASSIFLORA mother tincture in water before the evening meal.

Add one tablet of the chosen remedies in the morning and evening:

• After an emotional setback: GELSEMIUM 6C and IGNATIA 6C
• After an excessive workload: NUX VOMICA 6C
• After intellectual overexertion: KALI PHOSPHORICUM 6C
• After physical overexertion: ARNICA 6C and RHUS TOXICODENDRON 6C

• After worry which is not expressed: STAPHYSAGRIA 6C and AMBRA GRISEA 6C
• After sleepless nights (for example, looking after a sick person or revising for an exam): COCCULUS INDICUS 6C
• After a fright: ACONITE 6C
• After excessive consumption of food and/or alcohol: NUX VOMICA 6C
• After excessive consumption of coffee: COFFEA
• In a restless child: CHAMOMILLA 6C
• Fear of nightmares at the beginning of the night: BELLADONNA 6C and HYOSCYMUS 6C
• As a result of cramps: CUPRUM METALLICUM 6C
• Over-active mind, constantly thinking: COFFEA 6C
• During periods: CIMICIFUGA 6C

Chronic insomnia

People who suffer from chronic insomnia generally take sleeping tablets. It is therefore necessary to gradually wean them off these medicines by replacing them with constitutional remedies (chosen by a homeopath).

Warning

Avoid all sleeping pills, as they rapidly become habit-forming and can impair the memory and intellectual alertness.

Slimming

Homeopathy has no miracle cure for losing weight. Certain dubious slim-ming clinics use appetite suppressants, diuretics, and thyroid extracts.

However, a homeopath would be capable of helping you get slimmer if you were overweight by giving dietary advice and prescribing constitutional remedies. This problem can never be solved through self-medication.

Sneezing

See 'Colds'.

Sore throat

See 'Tonsillitis'.

Spices

See 'Cravings'.

Splinters

A splinter or thorn embedded in the skin may cause an infection. Once you have removed the foreign body, disinfect with a solution of CALENDULA (10 drops of mother tincture in a glass of water). Apply this twice a day, when you change the dressing. Then take LEDUM PALUSTRE 6C, ECHINACEA 6C, and HYPERICUM 6C, one tablet three times a day until the wound is healed.

Sprains

See 'Trauma and burns'.

Stiff joints

See 'Osteoarthritis'.

Stomach ache

See 'Digestive disorders'.

Storms

Some remedy types are aggravated by storms. These are RHODODENDRON, PHOSPHORUS, LACHESIS, and SEPIA.

Stress

See 'Nerves, fear, and anxiety'.

Stye

See 'The eye'.

Sunstroke

See 'Heat stroke'.

Surgical operations

See 'Trauma and burns'.

Sweating

Sweating is an essential function to regulate body temperature. Excessive sweating (or absence) or odour can cause concern. It is the expression of a person's general state of health, and thus will be noted by your homeopath when deciding on a constitutional remedy. However, problems can often be eased by self-medication.

You must not try to stop sweating, just to regulate it. It is fine to use a deodorant but not an anti-perspirant as the latter blocks the natural process of elimination. Homeopathic remedies act deeply, bringing back normal sweat patterns.

Take one tablet of the chosen remedies morning and night:

• For generalized or localized sweating in a jovial, active subject: SULPHUR 6C

• For sour-smelling head sweats, especially at night, particularly in infants: CALCAREA CARBONICA 6C

• For sweating in a baby while suckling: CALCAREA CARBONICA 6C

• For generalized sweating in an overweight person: CALCAREA CARBONICA 6C

• For generalized foul-smelling sweat: THUJA 6C

• For sweaty head and feet (with a bad smell): SILICA 6C

• For generalized or localized sweating in an emotional person prone to attacks of nerves: GELSEMIUM 6C

• For waking up covered in sweat: SAMBUCUS NIGRA 6C

• For sweating after a serious sickness, during convalescence: CHINA 6C.

• For sweating during periods: VERATRUM ALBUM 6C

Swollen stomach

See 'Digestive disorders'.

Teeth

Dental problems are often very painful. It is essential to maintain good oral hygiene and eat a healthy diet (not too much refined sugar!) to avoid a number of problems.

Only take the following remedies with the knowledge and consent of the treating dentist.

Dental abscess

MERCURIUS VIVUS 6C and FERRUM PHOSPHORICUM 6C, one tablet of each, every two hours.

Caries (tooth decay)

Take MEZERIUM 6C, KREOSOTUM 6C, and FLUORIC ACID 6C, one tablet of each, in the morning and evening during treatment. If the tooth is decayed down to the root, add THUJA 6C one tablet a day.

Dental extraction

• Preparation: ARNICA 6C and CHINA 6C, one tablet in the morning and evening in the preceding week

• After the extraction: mouthwash with a solution of 15 drops of HYPERCAL (a mixture of CALENDULA and HYPERICUM mother tinctures) in a little water, and take HYPERICUM 6C and MERCURIUS VIVUS 6C, one tablet of each twice a day.

Teething in babies

CHAMOMILLA 6C one tablet in the morning and evening and one tablet as needed for the pain.

Teething pains in toddlers

CALCAREA CARBONICA 6C and KREOSOTUM 6C, one tablet of each every morning and evening during teething.

Temper tantrums

See 'Behavioural problems'.

Tendonitis

See 'Joint pains'.

Thirst

The degree of thirst in a person is a guide to the choice of remedies:

• Permanent feeling of thirst with dry mouth: NATRUM MURIATICUM

• Absence of thirst despite fever: GELSEMIUM

• Absence of thirst despite a dry mouth: ALUMINA

• Extreme thirst for large quantities of water with a feeling of dryness in acute illnesses: BRYONIA

• Thirst for small amounts of cold water, which is then vomited: PHOSPHORUS and ARSENICUM ALBUM

Thrush

See 'The Mouth'.

Tinnitus

See 'Ringing in the ears'.

Tobacco

Tobacco causes numerous diseases: lung cancer, chronic bronchitis, chronic catarrh, asthma, cancer of the bladder, high blood pressure and cardiovascular disease. Giving up smoking is therefore common sense.

However, giving up smoking is not easy because it is highly addictive. Giving up smoking leads to an increased appetite and better absorption of food, which leads to weight gain. This, in itself, may cause a return to smoking.

It is necessary to see your homeopath for constitutional remedies to help you stop smoking. While awaiting this consultation, take NUX VOMICA 6C and ARGENTUM NITRICUM 6C, one tablet in the morning and evening and when there is a strong urge to smoke.

Acupuncture may be very useful in abolishing the cravings.

Tonsillitis

Inflammation of the tonsils may be caused by bacterial or viral infections. The throat can become sore even after the tonsils have been surgically removed.

The pain and swelling make it difficult to swallow.

Keep warm and gargle three or four times a day with warm water containing 15 drops of CALENDULA mother tincture.

• The throat is inflamed and red, swallowing is painful, the neck glands are slightly enlarged, and there is a fever of 100.4–102.2° F (38–39° C): BELLADONNA 6C and FERRUM PHOSPHORICUM 6C one tablet every 15 minutes until there is an improvement

• White spots appear at the back of the throat, the tongue is 'furred', the temperature rises: replace FERRUM PHOSPHORICUM with MERCURIUS VIVUS 6C

• If the pain is burning in nature and is improved by cold drinks, replace FERRUM PHOSPHORICUM with APIS MELLIFICA 6C

• If the throat is dry, swallowing difficult, and the pain spreads out to the ears, replace FERRUM PHOSPHORICA with PHYTOLACCA 6C

• If the throat is sore on the right, add LYCOPODIUM 6C, one tablet in the morning and evening

• If the throat is sore on the left, add LACHESIS 6C, one tablet in the morning and evening

Warning

Homeopathic treatment should calm the symptoms very quickly (in 24 hours); if this is not the case, consult a doctor, who will consider whether antibiotics are required.

Toothpaste

Contrary to the widely circulated rumour, all toothpastes are compatible with homeopathy, even those containing mint, and so everybody can use the toothpaste they like best, without any hesitation.

Torn muscle

ARNICA 6C, CHINA 6C and RHUS TOXICODENDRON 6C, one tablet of each, in the morning and evening will assist healing.

Trauma and burns

A medical examination is essential in all cases of trauma. Surgery may be required in certain cases.

Warning

Always make sure you clean a wound thoroughly to remove any foreign bodies. An X-ray may be needed to detect fragments of glass.

Burns

Only treat minor superficial burns at home. Full thickness or extensive burns require immediate medical attention.

Partial thickness burn

Take APIS MELLIFICA 6C, one tablet every 15 minutes. Add ARNICA 6C, if the skin looks purplish and feels bruised, or BELLADONNA 6C, if the skin is very red and the person is distressed.

If blistering occurs add RHUS TOXICODENDRON 6C, again one tablet every 15 minutes. If the blistering is more extensive, use CANTHARIS 6C instead of RHUS TOXICODENDRON.

Scars

To diminish thick, unsightly scars: GRAPHITES 6C, one tablet in the morning and evening. If they are red and purplish, add LACHESIS 6C and SULPHURIC ACID, at the same dose. If the scars are the result of a burn, add CAUSTICUM 6C.

Cuts

Disinfect with a solution of 15 drops of mother tincture CALENDULA in a little water, after washing the wound thoroughly with soap and water. Take STAPHYSAGRIA 6C and HYPERICUM 6C, one tablet morning and night, for two weeks.

Animal bites

Every bite must first be washed thoroughly with plenty of soap and water, and then covered with a compress of diluted CALENDULA. Rabies is virtually unknown in the United Kingdom, but it is a risk abroad, even in Europe. Preventative vaccination is available if there is a possibility of the disease.

To assist with wound healing, take the following combination: ARNICA 6C, LACHESIS 6C, and LEDUM PALUSTRE 6C for two weeks.

Insect bites and stings

All insect bites (bees, wasps, mosquitoes etc.) are helped by homeopathic remedies: APIS MELLIFICA 6C and LEDUM PALUSTRE 6C: one tablet of each every 15 minutes, decreasing the frequency as you notice an improvement.

Traumas in general

The use of homeopathy in trauma provides the best evidence base for its efficiency. ARNICA 6C stands out as being exceptionally useful.

After a trauma, take one tablet of ARNICA 6C every hour, together with a remedy chosen for its specific action; decrease the frequency when you notice an improvement.

- For bruises: HAMAMELIS 6C
- For a pulled muscle: CHINA 6C
- For sprains: RUTA 6C and RHUS TOXICODENDRON 6C
- For fractures: SYMPHYTUM 6C and CALCAREA PHOSPHORICA 6C

- For the eyes: HAMAMELIS 6C and LEDUM PALUSTE 6C
- For the nerves: HYPERICUM 6C
- For the breasts: BELLIS PERENNIS 6C
- For the skull: NATRUM SULPHURICUM 6C

Travel sickness

Whatever the mode of transport, take one tablet of each remedy every hour throughout the journey: COCCULUS 6C, TABACUM 6C, GELSEMIUM 6C, and PETROLEUM 6C.

Traveller's diarrhoea

See 'Colic' and 'Diarrhoea'.

Tremor

A consultation with your doctor and possibly a neurologist is essential to diagnose the cause of tremor.

For tremors caused by anxiety, take: GELSEMIUM 6C, ARGENTUM NITRICUM 6C, and IGNATIA 6C, one tablet of each remedy in the morning and evening, and when gripped by strong emotions.

Uterine fibroids

See 'Female reproductive system'.

Urinary incontinence

See 'Bedwetting'.

Homeopathy encyclopedia

Urinary infection

See 'Cystitis'.

Urticaria

See 'Skin, hair, and nails'.

Vaccinations (prevention of side effects)

All vaccines disrupt the equilibrium of the body. To combat these side effects, take THUJA 30C the night before, the day of vaccination, and the following day.

Vaginal discharge

See 'Female reproductive system'.

Vaginismus

A painful spasm of the vagina making sexual intercourse impossible, usually it has a psychological basis and thus responds well to counselling. Homeopathic remedies are helpful additional therapy.

Take one tablets of the chosen remedy in the morning and evening, according to the situation:

• For a very sensitive and emotional woman: IGNATIA 6C

• When vaginismus appears after first sexual experience: STAPHYSAGRIA 6C

• For increased sensitivity of the vagina: BERBERIS 6C

Varicose ulcer

A skin wound developing in association with varicose veins requires a great deal of care and attention and should be seen by a doctor. A homeopath can prescribe suitable remedies.

Wash the area with diluted CALENDULA (10 drops of mother tincture in a glass of water) and while waiting for constitutional treatment, take:

• If the ulcer is painless or only slightly painful: AESCULUS HIPPOCASTRUM 6C, FLUORIC ACID 6C, and KALI BICHROMICUM 6C, one tablet of each three times a day

• If the ulcer is very painful: HEPAR SULPH 6C, LACHESIS 6C, and ARSENICUM ALBUM 6C, one tablet of each, three times a day

Varicose veins

Varicose veins are permanently dilated veins. Only surgery will remove them. They can cause the feeling of 'heavy legs'. Physical exercise, particularly walking, is an excellent way to prevent the development of varicose veins.

Homeopathic remedies can help to slow down the development of varicose disease and reduce the risks of complications such as phlebitis (inflammation) and varicose ulcers.

Take AESCULUS HIPPOCASTRUM 6C, ARNICA 6C, and HAMAMELIS 6C, one tablet of each remedy twice a day, and FLUORIC ACID 6C once a day.

When there is a danger of phlebitis, take: LACHESIS 6C and VIPERA 6C and see the doctor immediately.

Warning

Avoid traumas to a varicose vein as a varicose ulcer may result.

Varicosities (spider veins)

These small, dilated blood vessels are particularly found on the lower limbs and face. Use the same treatment as for varicose veins (see above).

Veins

The veins are vessels that allow the blood to return to the heart. Unlike the arteries, they have no muscle in their walls and can become dilated. Varicose veins appear when this distension becomes irreversible. It is therefore advisable to treat them as soon as any problem comes to your notice.

For heaviness and pain along the course of the veins: AESCULUS HIPPOCASTANUM 6C, ARNICA 6C, and HAMAMELIS 6C, one tablet of each in the morning and evening, for two weeks.

Voice loss

The voice may be totally lost or become weak and hoarse. If this persists or is recurrent see your doctor as soon as possible. Do not force your voice, as this will only make matters worse.

Take one tablet every hour on the first day, then three times a day on the following days:

• For singers and public speakers: ARNICA 6C, ARUM TRIPHYLLUM 6C, and ARGENTUM NITRICUM 6C

• After excessive shouting or singing: ARNICA 6C and RHUS TOXICODEN-DRON 6C

• After getting cold: ACONITE 6C and ARUM TRIPHYLLUM 6C

• After a fright or emotional shock: GELSEMIUM 6C and AMMONIUM CARBONICUM 6C

Warning

Consult a doctor or homeopath if the symptoms do not subside in 48 hours.

Vomiting

See 'Digestive problems'.

Warts

See 'Skin, hair, and nails'.

Weight loss

Weight loss without any other obvious symptoms always requires a medical

Homeopathy encyclopedia

consultation to find the cause. If investigations fail to find a cause, take:

• Adolescents: NATRUM MURIATICUM 6C and CALCAREA PHOSPHORICA 6C, one tablet twice a day

• Adults: SILICA 6C, one tablet twice a day

Whitlow

A whitlow is an infection on a finger or toe, near the nail, that must be treated in the same way as an abscess. However, you can also add two remedies that will slow down its progress: MYRISTICA 6C and ECHINACEA 6C, one tablet of each three times a day.

See 'Abscesses and boils'.

Whooping cough

This is a highly contagious bacterial infection particularly found in children aged from two to seven. It is rare nowadays due to vaccination. It can lead to serious complications and you must see the doctor immediately if you suspect it. Homeopathic remedies can be helpful to ease the troublesome cough; seek professional advice.

Worms

Worm infection is common in small children, causing itchiness around the anus. Try CINA 6C and TEUCRIUM MARUM 6C, one tablet of each, twice a day. If this does not clear the infestation, consult your doctor.

Wounds

See 'Traumas and burns'.

3
Remedies

Abies nigra

Source of the remedy
The resin of the black spruce, Abies nigra

Main actions
Spasms of the stomach

Modalities
Aggravation with coffee and tea

Site of action
The digestive tract

Related remedies

Ignatia, Thuja, and Nux Vomica

Abrotanum

Source of the remedy
The fresh leaves and stems of the Artemisia abrotanum plant

Main actions
Malnutrition, weight loss, diarrhoea with significant fluid loss

Secondary signs
Rheumatism following diarrhoea. Alternating diarrhoea and rheumatism

Suggested uses
1. Malnutrition with severe weight loss

2. Gout and rheumatism

3. Chilblains and Raynaud's syndrome

Site of action
• The general health

• The joints

• The small blood vessels

Related remedies

Natrum muriaticum, Veratrum album, China, Arsenicum album and, Secale cornutum

Aconite napellus

Aconite in brief
• An emergency remedy

• At the onset of all inflammatory conditions (colds, sore throats, laryngitis, bronchitis, pleurisy)

• Cardiovascular system

• Excitement of the nervous system

Source of the remedy
The whole Monkshood plant

Main actions
Excitement, anxiety and fear of death; neuralgia; rapid heart rate with a strong pulse; congestion, hypertension (high blood pressure), and haemorrhage

Modalities
• Aggravated at night (after midnight), made worse by a cold snap, by lying on the painful side

• Better for sweating

Suggested uses
1. At the onset of all feverish conditions, whatever the cause: colds, sore throats, laryngitis, bronchitis, pleurisy, pneumonia, rheumatism (especially following a cold snap). Aconite is no longer useful once sweating occurs

2. Acute elevation of the blood pressure in an anxious person

3. Acute neuralgia

4. Acute anxiety attacks

5. Periods that stop following a cold snap

Site of action
• The immune system

• The nervous system

• The cardiovascular system

Related remedies

Belladonna and Ferrum phosphoricum

Sensitive type

Aconite gives the best results in young, energetic people

Actea racemosa
See Cimicifuga, another name for the remedy.

Actea spicata
Source of the remedy
The roots of the Baneberry plant

Main actions
Rheumatism with deformity; nodules and pain in the wrists, hands, and fingers; painful swelling of the limbs

Modalities
Aggravated by movement, the damp cold, and being touched

Site of action
The joints, particularly small joints

Related remedies

Ruta, Natrum carbonicum, Sepia, Sulphur iodatum, Caulophyllum, and Lycopodium

Aesculus hippocastanum
Aesculus in brief
A wonderful remedy for congestion of the veins, especially haemorrhoids.

Source of the remedy
The Horse Chestnut kernel

Main actions
Congestion especially in the liver and pelvis, with haemorrhoids and pelvic congestion. Pain in the lumbar area, especially around the sacro-iliac area

Secondary signs
Feelings of heaviness and fullness in the pelvis; a prickling sensation in the rectum

Modalities
• Aggravated by sleep, waking up and heat

• Better for cold, moderate exercise

Suggested uses
1. Haemorrhoids which bleed slightly, in a person with venous congestion

2. Pelvic congestion

3. Varicose veins and varicose ulcers

4. Congestive headaches

5. Congestive conjunctivitis

Site of action
The veins

Related remedies

Arnica, Hamamelis, and Sepia

Sensitive Type

Slow, passive individuals.

Aethusa cynapium
Source of the remedy
Fool's Parsley, the whole plant in bloom

Main actions
Gastro-enteritis; convulsions in infants; milk intolerance; dehydration; collapse

Modalities
• Aggravated by milk, the cold, and during teething

Suggested uses
1. Gastro-enteritis in infants with immediate vomiting, refusal to drink, and severe weakness

2. Cholera in an adult

3. Lack of concentration in school children

Site of action
• The digestive system

• The central nervous system

Related remedies

Chamomilla, Ipecac, Veratrum album, and Abrotanum

Agaricus muscarius
Agaricus in brief
• Muscular spasms, tics, and trembling

• Chilblains

• Intoxication with alcohol

Source of the remedy
The Fly Agaric mushroom

Main actions
Severe diarrhoea; excitation resembling drunkenness; delirium, hallucinations, spasms, trembling, convulsions, and involuntary muscular contractions; itchy red rashes with a pricking sensation and ice-like coldness

Modalities
• Worse for sex, excessive study, and the cold

• Better for sleep and gentle movement

Suggested uses
1. Tics and muscular spasms in children, especially when they are tired

2. Trembling in the senile

3. Itching, burning chilblains

4. Alcoholic intoxication

5. Spasmodic eye movements

6. Intellectual weakness

Site of action
• The muscular system

• The central nervous system

Agnus castus

Agnus castus in brief
Action on the libido

Source of the remedy
The berries of a small tree, the Chaste tree.

Main actions
Low sexual function in both men and women, with a low libido. Intense depression with a lack of energy

Secondary signs
Breast milk production

Suggested uses
1. Impotence and frigidity without sexual desire

2. Lack of breast milk in a woman who has recently given birth

Site of action
The reproductive systems of both men and women

Related remedies

Selenium

Agraphis nutans

Source of the remedy
The whole Bluebell plant

Main actions
Tonsillitis; inflammation of the adenoids; catarrh with tonsillitis

Modalities
• Aggravated by the cold

Site of action
The immune system

Related remedies

Baryta carbonica and Calcarea carbonica

Ailanthus glandulosa

Source of the remedy
The leaves and growing shoots of the 'Tree of heaven'

Main actions
Throat infections and infective ulcers of the tonsils; pharyngitis; severe infections; scarlet fever; remedy to be used alongside antibiotics

Site of action
The immune system

Related remedies

Lachesis, Mercurius cyanatus, and Pyrogen

Aletris farinosa

Source of the remedy
The dried root of the Stargrass plant

Main actions
Great fatigue after periods, vaginal discharge, and bleeding between periods. Constipation, without desire to open the bowels and with great straining at stool

Site of action
• The female reproductive system

• The intestines

Related remedies

Alumina, Lycopodium, and Silica

Alfalfa

Source of the remedy
The whole Californian Clover plant, when in bloom

Main actions
Physical and emotional debility with sadness and nervousness. Insomnia after mental overexertion

Site of action
The general health

Related remedies

Avena sativa

Allium cepa

Allium cepa in brief
Remedy for acute ear, nose, and throat complaints

Source of the remedy
The Red Onion

Main actions
Irritation of the whole respiratory system; abdominal colic with gas; painful inflammation of the sensory nerves; irritation of the conjunctiva

Secondary signs
Burning, irritating, watery nasal discharge, leading to redness of the nose and upper lip; non-irritant watery eyes; frequent sneezing; hoarse, spasmodic cough with a searing pain in the larynx (windpipe)

Suggested uses
1. Colds and flu

2. Hay fever

Related remedies

Euphrasia

Allium sativa

Source of the remedy
The Garlic Bulb

Main actions
Heaviness in the stomach, painful abdominal distension, foul-smelling wind, and abdominal colic in big eaters, especially meat eaters. High blood pressure in ruddy individuals

Site of action
• The digestive system

• The cardiovascular system

Related remedies

Sulphur, Nux vomica, and Antimonium crudum

Aloe socotrina

Source of the remedy
The sap from the leaves of the Common Aloe plant

Main actions
Irritation of the intestines with burning diarrhoea and haemorrhoids, with faecal incontinence in heavy meat eaters. Headaches. Intellectual laziness

Modalities
• Aggravated by waking, after meals, the heat, and drinking beer

• Haemorrhoids better for cold baths

Site of action
The digestive system

Related remedies

Sulphur, Nux vomica, Podophyllum, and Aesculus

Alumina

Alumina in brief
Remedy for prematurely old people with dehydration, and slowing of the metabolism and digestion

Source of the remedy
Alumina, the oxide of aluminium

Main actions
Mental fatigue with depression. Dryness of the digestive tract with slow digestion. General dehydration with wrinkled skin and premature ageing. Fatigue

Secondary signs
Paralysis, especially of the eyes; vertigo; suicidal tendencies

Modalities
• Aggravated by cold, dry weather, and in the mornings

• Better for fresh air and cold water

Suggested uses
1. Constipation with slow digestion

2. Dry mouth without thirst. Dehydration

3. Slow thought processes with anxiety

Related remedies

Lycopodium, Silica, and Bryonia.

Ambra grisea

Ambra grisea in brief
• Emotional hypersensitivity

• Tics and nervous spasms

• Depression

Source of the remedy
Ambergris, the secretion of the sperm whale

Main actions
Emotional hypersensitivity

Marked spasms

Blood vessel fragility with a tendency to haemorrhage

Secondary signs
Insomnia; muscular cramps, spasmodic cough, and constipation with cramps; itching of the genitals; bleeding between periods

Modalities
• Aggravated by music and when in company

• Better for cold air, cold drinks, and cold food

Suggested uses
1. Emotional hypersensitivity with loss of consciousness

2. Attacks of nerves

3. Bleeding between periods

4. Spasms of every organ

5. Depression and premature senility

Homeopathy encyclopedia

Related remedies

Ignatia, Gelsemium, and Pulsatilla

Ammonium carbonicum

Ammonium carbonicum in brief

• Remedy for blocked noses

• Asthma with attacks in the middle of the night

Source of the remedy

Ammonium carbonate

Main actions

Thick, irritating secretions from the digestive and respiratory systems, with difficulty in expectoration. Haemorrhages of black blood from the nose, the bowels, and the uterus, and a tendency to kidney problems

Secondary signs

Cold with a blocked nose, worse at 2 to 3a.m.; swelling of the gums

Modalities

• Worse at 4 a.m.

• Aggravated by physical exertion, in a warm room

• Better for sleeping on the stomach

Suggested uses

1. Colds with blocked nose and nosebleeds

2. Asthma at 3 a.m.

3. Emphysema and bronchitis in the elderly

Site of action

The lining of the respiratory system and the nose

Related remedies

Kali carbonicum

Ammonium muriaticum

Ammonium muriaticum in brief

• Remedy for colds with abundant secretions and loss of sense of smell

• Constipation

Source of the remedy

Ammonium chloride

Main actions

The opposite of Ammonium carbonicum: increased secretions, clear and abundant

Secondary signs

Colds with sneezing and irritation of the lip; loss of the senses of smell and taste; obstinate constipation with gas; hard stools, difficult to pass with burning in the rectum and anus; sciatic pains

Modalities

• Aggravated by the cold and walking

• Sciatica worse for sitting and better for lying down

Suggested uses

1. Colds with copious secretions

2. Constipation

3. Sciatica and rheumatism

Sites of action
• The linings of the respiratory system: nose, throat, and bronchi

• The intestines

• The nerves

Related remedies

Pulsatilla

Amyl nitrate

Amyl nitrate in brief
Remedy for conditions caused by dilated blood vessels

Source of the remedy
Amyl nitrate

Main actions
Acute remedy for congestion of the head, with dilation of the blood vessels, redness and intense heat in the face and whole body. Increased awareness of the heartbeat, without any increase in the pulse rate

Secondary signs
Violent beating of the neck arteries and the heart. Headache, throbbing of the temples with no increase in the blood pressure

Suggested uses
1. Acute conditions caused by dilated blood vessels

2. Headaches, hot flushes, and pounding heart

Anacardium orientale

Anacardium orientale in brief
• Intellectual fatigue
• Headache

Source of the remedy
The Marking nut

Main actions
Loss of memory, depression, and split personality; delusions of persecution; hallucinations, especially of the sense of smell; headaches; stomach and duodenal pains relieved by eating

Secondary signs
Intellectual fatigue in a person with a difficult character; headaches in students; loss of memory; bulimia in obese people

Site of action
The central nervous system

Related remedies
Kali phosphoricum

Sensitive type

An intellectual, a student, or an adult, with nervous exhaustion and a strange feeling of having a dual personality

Anagallis arvensis
Source of the remedy
The whole Scarlet Pimpernel plant

Main actions
Itchy blisters on the palms and soles

Site of action
• The skin
• The immune system

Homeopathy encyclopedia

Angustura vera

Source of the remedy
The bark of the Galipea cusparia tree

Main actions
Contractions, and painful stiffness in the joints, especially the knees; cramps; tendonitis

Site of action
The muscles and joints

Related remedies

Rhus toxicodendron, Ruta, Cimicifuga, and Cuprum metallicum

Antimonium crudum

Antimonium crudum in brief
• Overeating in greedy people

• Blistering or pustular rashes

• Warts with horny patches

Source of the remedy
Black Sulphide of Antimony

Main actions
Irritation of the digestive tract, particularly the stomach. Rashes, and severe thickening of the skin

Secondary signs
Craving for acidic food and drink, even though it is badly tolerated

Modalities
• Aggravated by cold baths and by radiant heat

• Improved by hot baths, resting, and open air

Suggested uses
1. Overeating with a thick, white, 'furred' tongue with a thick coat, belching, nausea, vomiting that provides no relief, diarrhoea

2. Rashes of blisters or pustules, with a tendency to impetigo

3. Hard, horny warts

Site of action
• The central nervous system (heat regulation, control of appetite)

• The digestive system

• The skin

Related remedies

Nux vomica and Nitric acid (warts)

Sensitive type

• Fat, greedy child or adult

• Grumpy person with skin infections

Antimonium tartaricum

Antimonium tartaricum in brief
• Remedy for chest complaints with thick secretions

• Certain types of acne

Source of the remedy
Tartrate of Antimony and Potash

Main actions
Accumulation of thick, abundant secretions, especially in the small wind pipes. Exhaustion, pallor, sleepiness, and weakness

Secondary signs
Craving for acid food (fruit) that upset; aversion to milk; smallpox-type rashes

Modalities
• Aggravated by damp cold, the heat of the room, and lying down

• Improved by fresh air, expectoration, and a sitting position

Suggested uses
1. Acute or chronic lung disorders with difficulty in expectorating and a tendency to asphyxia: bronchitis, asthma, and emphysema

2. Pustular acne

3. Constant nausea with considerable anxiety

Site of action
• The respiratory system

• The central nervous system

• The skin

Related remedies

Ipecac

Apis mellifica
Apis mellifica in brief
• Emergency remedy for sudden swelling, particularly after insect bites

• Remedy for fluid in chest, around the heart, in the abdomen, in joints, and around the brain

Source of the remedy
The whole Bee

Main actions
Swellings that appear suddenly, with burning and stinging pains

Secondary signs
The skin is dry or slightly sweaty; accumulations of fluid in an organ

Modalities
• Aggravated by heat, being touched, and pressure

• Improved by cold, the open air

Suggested uses
1. Any swelling that appears suddenly, wherever it is located

2. Insect bites

3. Sunstroke

4. Urticaria

5. Fluid in the lung lining (pleurisy), around the heart (pericarditis), the brain coverings (meningitis), or a joint

6. The early stages of boils and whitlows

7. Kidney failure

Site of action
• The membranes

• The skin

• The kidneys

Related remedies

Ledum palustre and Bryonia

Aralia racemosa
Aralia racemosa in brief
Remedy for allergic rhinitis and asthma at the beginning of the night

Homeopathy encyclopedia

Source of the remedy
The root of the plant known as American Spikenard

Main actions
Rhinitis with copious irritating watery discharge and sneezing

Secondary signs
Spasmodic cough

Modalities
• Aggravated by lying down before 11 p.m., draughts, and cold

Suggested uses
1. Allergic rhinitis with a spasmodic cough that appears when the subject lies down, or around 11 p.m.

2. Asthma with a spasmodic cough

Site of action
The respiratory system

Related remedies

Lachesis and Hyoscyamus

Aranea diadema
Source of the remedy
The Papal Cross Spider, used whole and alive

Main actions
Neuralgia and bone pains that occur at regular intervals; facial neuralgia; night-time shoulder pains; sensory disorders

Modalities
• Aggravated by humidity

Site of action
The central nervous system

Related remedies

Cedron, Arsenicum album, and China

Argentum metallicum
Source of the remedy
The metal, Silver

Main actions
Laryngitis and painful chronic inflammations of the pharynx, especially in singers; greyish mucous phlegm

Site of action
The larynx

Related remedies

Argentum nitricum, often used instead

Argentum nitricum
Argentum nitricum in brief
• Major remedy for nervous conditions

• Very painful laryngitis

Source of the remedy
Silver Nitrate

Main actions
Anxiety; nervous anticipation; a compulsion to hurry

Secondary signs
Fatigue from overexertion; trembling, vertigo caused by heights; inflammation of the digestive tract and the genital organs with occasional ulceration, and the sensation of a trapped splinter; craving for sweet food; prolonged belching after meals

Modalities

- Aggravated by all forms of heat, during periods, by sweet food

- Improved by cold or cool weather, by heavy pressure

Suggested uses

1. Nervous anticipation in a restless, anxious, overworked subject

2. Headaches improved by pressure

3. Conjunctivitis, laryngitis, pharyngitis with the feeling of a splinter lodged in the throat, and constant clearing of the throat

4. Stomach pains with wind, swelling, and belching. Stomach ulcers

5. Emotional diarrhoea

6. Inflammatory bowel diseases

Site of action

- The nervous system

- The membranes of the digestive and respiratory systems

Related remedies

Gelsemium

Sensitive type

Thin, despondent, prematurely aged subject, always restless, anxious, in a hurry, and prone to nerves. Fear of heights and a tendency to vertigo

Aristolochia clemantis

Source of the remedy

The flowering Aristolochia plant

Main actions

Light periods, late periods, or absence of periods; nervousness before and after periods; cold limbs; poor circulation; varicose veins

Modalities

- Worse before and after periods

- Better during periods, by cool air, by movement

Site of action

- The female reproductive system

- The veins

Related remedies

Pulsatilla

Arnica montana

Arnica in brief

- An emergency remedy

- For all physical trauma

- The cardiovascular system

- Depressions after a psychological shock

- Serious high fevers with restlessness

Source of the remedy

The whole Arnica plant, when in flower

Main actions

Pain and stiffness in the muscles; bruising; overexertion; fever with a lack of energy

Secondary signs

Psychological shocks; depression; despair after a challenge; overwork

Arnica montana

Modalities
• Worse for the slightest touch, movement, and damp weather

• Improved by rest, by lying down

Suggested uses
1. All trauma: post-operative, post-natal (for both mother and child), minor haemorrhages, all blows, falls, and accidents, overworked hearts in sports competitors, hoarseness in singers or public speakers, the effects of strenuous work and long walks

2. Serious fevers whatever the cause. There is restlessness, aversion to touch, shivering, and extreme thirst. The face is red and congested, the nose and the rest of the body are cold. The breath is foetid. Bruises appear

3. Anxious depressions with intense fatigue and fear of death

Site of action
• The cardiovascular system

• The nervous system

• The emotional state

Sensitive type

The Arnica subject is often a great sports player and is always active. He or she is somewhat taciturn, dislikes physical contact, is quick to display irritation or sadness, and is often plagued by nightmares.

Arsenicum album
Arsenicum album in brief
• Major remedy (polychrest)

• For serious health conditions

• Acute infections

• Mania and obsessive personality

• Allergies (asthma and eczema)

• Periodically recurring diseases

Source of the remedy
The oxide of Arsenic

Main actions
Ulceration of all the membranes; serious diseases of the kidneys, liver, and adrenals; serious diseases of the nervous system: paralysis, convulsions, and coma

Secondary signs
Progressive decline in all the vital body functions; cramps and trembling; dry skin with hardening and scaly rashes; burning pains improved by heat; burning, aggressive, acrid, foul-smelling secretions; frequent thirst for small amounts of cold water; combination of anxiety, restlessness, and weakness; sensitivity to cold; nausea at the sight or smell of food

Modalities
• Aggravation between 1 and 3 a.m., from the cold, from ice-cold food and drinks, from being face down

• Improved by heat of all kinds (except headaches), from hot food and drink, from changes in position

Suggested uses
• Acute indications:

1. Serious infections

2. Severe acute gastro-enteritis, food poisoning

3. Acute cystitis

4. Inflammations of the womb and vagina

5. Burning neuralgic pains aggravated by heat

6. Asthma, head colds and hay fever, alternating with skin rashes

7. Acute, burning skin infections: boils, carbuncles

• Chronic indications:

1. Recurrent complaints: asthma, hay fever, chronic skin diseases such as dry eczema, anxiety states, weakness, depression

2. Great susceptibility to parasites

3. Long convalescence after a disease

Sites of action
• The immune system

• All the major organs

• The skin

• The emotional state

Related remedies

Psorinum and Tuberculinum koch

Sensitive type

A precise, thrifty individual, who is meticulous often to the point of extreme fussiness. Life is viewed as a ritual, governed by well-established rules. Both morally and physically, he or she is 'dressed up to the nines'. There is permanent anxiety and, frequently, an irrational fear of dying. Often thin and lanky, he or she has a pale complexion but a piercing gaze. A remarkable technician, or a shrewd administrator, often one of the cornerstones of a company. This is a person who suffers with allergies, asthma and eczema, and is very frightened of asthma attacks. When he or she falls sick, a truly obsessive tidiness sets in.

Arsenicum iodatum
Source of the remedy
Iodide of Arsenic

Main actions
Burning rhinitis with a tendency to become chronic; weakness, restlessness, weight loss; weakness of the heart with disturbances of the heart rhythm; bronchitis; asthma

Secondary signs
Swollen glands with increased thyroid activity (hyperthyroidism); scaling of the skin in large patches

Modalities
• Aggravated by eating

• Improved by cold and heat

Suggested uses
1. Allergic rhinitis

2. Asthma

3. Profound weakness with restlessness and anxiety

4. A weak heart in elderly people

5. Certain types of eczema

Sites of action
• The immune system

• The heart and lungs

• The skin

Related remedies

Kali iodatum, Iodum, Natrum muriaticum and Tuberculinum

Artemisia vulgaris
Source of the remedy
The root of the Mugwort plant

Main actions
Epileptic fits, particularly in puberty. Note that this remedy cannot replace the classical allopathic remedies. Convulsions and trembling in young subjects

Site of action
The central nervous system

Arum triphyllum
Source of the remedy
The dried root of the Jack-in-the-Pulpit plant

Main actions
Inflammation of the linings of the nose, pharynx, and larynx, which turn bright red. Irritation of the nostrils and the upper lip, to such an extent that they bleed

Suggested uses
1. Acute inflammation of the nose and pharynx, with bleeding

2. Laryngitis with very painful loss of voice, especially in singers

3. Seasonal allergic laryngitis

Sites of action
• The nose, pharynx and larynx

• The immune system

Related remedies

Belladonna

Asafoetida
Source of the remedy
The gum of the root of the Stinkasand plant

Main actions
Stomach wind with spasms; convulsions; spasms in all the muscles; increased muscular sensitivity, heightened reflexes, sensory disorders; wind and spasms in the oesophagus, making it impossible to swallow

Modalities
• Aggravated by the slightest touch and at night

• Improved in the open air and by the slightest movement

Site of action
The nervous system

Related remedies

Ignatia, Gelsemium and Argentum nitricum

Asarum

Source of the remedy
The root of the European Snake-Root plant

Main actions
Intolerably hypersensitive hearing; intolerance of noise, especially in alcoholics

Site of action
The central nervous system

Related remedies

Lachesis, Aurum, and Theridion

Asclepias tuberosa

Source of the remedy
The roots of the Butterfly Weed plant

Main actions
Chest pains on the left side which are triggered by dry pleurisy or vertebral problems

Site of action
The nerves

Related remedies

Natrum sulphuricum, Kali carbonicum and Dulcamara

Asterias rubens

Source of the remedy
The starfish used whole

Main actions
Painful benign tumours in the breasts, especially on the left-hand side (mastitis)

A remedy for breast cancer, but only as a complement to allopathic treatment

Site of action
• The breasts

• The immune system

Related remedies

Bryonia, Conium, Phytolacca, and Thuja.

Aurum metallicum

Aurum metallicum in brief
• Major remedy (polychrest)

• For high blood pressure

• Suicidal depression

• Rheumatism and bone pains

Source of the remedy
The metal gold

Main actions
Depression, world-weariness; tendency to high blood pressure, congestion, fast heart rate; tendency to swelling and hardening of the glands and lymphatic tissues; tooth decay; sensitivity to cold

Secondary signs
Suicidal tendency; swelling and hardening of the testicles; pains in the bones and joints; inflammatory rheumatism with intense pains at night that penetrate right into the bones

Homeopathy encyclopedia

Modalities

• Aggravated at night, by cold, in winter, by noise, alcohol, and intellectual overload

• Improved in summer, by heat and localized coolness, and by music

Suggested uses

1. High blood pressure with excess weight. Angina with extra heart beats

2. Infections and suppurations in the ears, nose, and throat

3. Deep-seated dental infections affecting the bone, with gland swelling

4. Inflammatory rheumatism

5. Depression in obese subjects with high blood pressure

Sites of action

• The arteries

• The emotional state, tendency to depression

• The skeletal system

Related remedies

Arsenicum album and Nux vomica

Sensitive type

Just like gold, these people are brilliant, as well as being expansive, warm, hard working, dominating, and sometimes violent to the point of tyranny. They are hypersensitive and constantly doubting themselves and the purpose of what they are undertaking. A great flexibility allows them to integrate easily into new situations.

They are leaders and builders, thirsty for knowledge and action; they may be engineers responsible for large-scale building projects or directors of major research programmes.

These subjects are often muscular, obese, and ruddy-faced. They are lively, boisterous, and restless, with a great need to expend physical energy.

Aurum muriaticum natronatum/Aurum muriaticum kalinatum

Source of the remedy

The salts of Gold: Sodium Tetrachloroaurate and Potassium Chloroaurate

Main actions

Action on uterine fibroids. Aurum muriaticum natronatum is suitable if the fibroid does not have a tendency to bleed, while Aurum muriaticum kalinatum should be chosen if it does

Site of action

The uterus

Related remedies

Thuja, Conium, and Lapis albus

Avena sativa

Avena sativa in brief

A fortifying remedy

Source of the remedy

The Common Oat

Main actions
A very good little remedy, a fortifying tonic to be used at 3x or 4x in all types of fatigue with a loss of appetite, after infectious diseases, and in cases of learning difficulties and poor concentration at school

Site of action
• The general health

• The immune system

Related remedies

Silica and Kali carbonicum

Badiaga

Source of the remedy
A dried Freshwater Sponge

Main actions
Swollen, inflamed, and painful lymph nodes; exophthalmic goitre (thyroid swelling with prominent, bulging eyes); allergic laryngitis with a troublesome cough; whooping cough

Modalities
• Aggravated by cold and stormy weather

Site of action
• The immune system

• The thyroid gland

Related remedies

Iodum and Sambucus

Baptisia tinctoria

Source of the remedy
The roots of the Wild Indigo

Main actions
Pharyngitis, diarrhoea, and fever with delirium; remedy used for serious infections, as a complement to classical treatment, particularly antibiotics

Site of action
• The immune system

Related remedies

Arsenicum album, Arnica, and Lachesis

Baryta carbonica

Remedy for intellectual retardation and enlarged lymph glands

Source of the remedy
Barium carbonate

Main actions
Physical and psychological retardation; intellectual slowness; atherosclerosis and high blood pressure; enlarged tonsils and benign prostate enlargement; great sensitivity to cold

Secondary signs
Aggravated by the slightest cold

Suggested uses
• Backwardness in school

• Retardation of physical and intellectual development

• Enlargement of the tonsils

• High blood pressure due to atherosclerosis

• Benign prostate enlargement

Baryta carbonica

Site of action
• The central nervous system

• The lymphatic system

• The endocrine glands

Sensitive type

A child who is behind in everything, and easily frightened by strangers

Belladonna
Belladona in brief
Emergency remedy
• Congestion

• Inflammation

• Hypersensitivity

• Excitability

Source of the remedy
Atropa Belladonna, the whole flowering Deadly Nightshade plant

Main actions
High fever with a drop in the pulse rate; dryness of the membranes; exhaustion; violent delirium; paralysis; coma and death

Secondary signs
Symptoms appear suddenly and with great violence; intense congestion and general and localized irritations with redness, heat, swelling, and pain; throbbing arteries; spasms

Modalities
• Aggravated by the slightest external influence: noise, bright light, cold,

draughts of air, being touched or shaken

• Improved by rest and heat

Suggested uses
1. All ailments with a sudden, violent onset

2. All intense general or localized congestion

3. All infectious diseases in adults or children with: flushed red face, temperature fluctuating wildly in the range 102.2–104° F/39–40° C, hot sweats, throbbing headaches, sometimes exhaustion and delirium

4. All local diseases with shiny red face, swellings that appear suddenly, throbbing pain, radiating heat, like the beginning of an abscess

5. Tonsillitis. Dry cough

Site of action
• The immune system during infectious diseases

• All inflammatory conditions

Related remedies

Aconite, Apis mellifica, Ferrum phosphoricum, Gelsemium, and Stramonium

Sensitive type

Close to that of Sulphur charming and very convivial when in good health, irritable and aggressive when sick. This remedy works well in Calcarea carbonica subjects.

Bellis perennis

Bellis perennis in brief
Remedy for all traumas

Source of the remedy
The Daisy, whole and in bloom

Main actions
Close to that of Arnica (see Arnica)

Suggested uses
With Arnica, in cases of trauma to the breast and the pelvis

Related remedies

Arnica

Benzoic acid

Benzoic acid in brief
Remedy for attacks of gout and for kidney stones

Source of the remedy
Benzoic acid

Main actions
Irritation of the bladder; joint pains that move from one place to another; palpitations that occur regularly around 2 a.m.

Secondary signs
Sparse, dark urine with a strong smell; stones in the urinary system

Modalities
• Aggravated around 2 a.m.

• Improved by increased urination

Suggested uses
1. Attacks of gout

2. Kidney stones

3. Inflammation of the prostate gland

4. Palpitations at night

Site of action
• The urinary system

• The joints

Related remedies

Berberis vulgaris

Sensitive type

Rheumatic person with a tendency to gout and kidney stones. The joint pains are more severe when the urinary flow is reduced.

Berberis vulgaris

Berberis vulgaris in brief
• Emergency and drainage remedy

• For drainage of the kidneys and liver

• Gallstones and kidney stones with colic

• Gout and rheumatism

Source of the remedy
The bark of the dried root of the Barberry shrub

Main actions
Reduction in urine output, red sediment in the urine; pain in the low back, especially on the left side, that spreads out as it goes down; kidney stones; gallbladder colic; attacks of gout

Secondary signs
Itchy, irritated red skin; burning, stinging pains that constantly change posi-

Homeopathy encyclopedia

tion and spread out extensively; 'bubbling' feeling in the kidney area

Modalities

• Aggravated by movement and jolts

• Improved by resting and after a good urine output

Suggested uses

1. Kidney and liver problems in people with a big appetite, pain in the gallbladder area, constipation or diarrhoea, haemorrhages and anal fissures

2. Kidney stones with colic, especially on the left-hand side, and variable urine output

3. Attacks of gout or rheumatism

4. Burning, itchy rashes on the back of the hands and in the anus

Site of action

• The liver and kidneys

• The joints

• The skin

Related remedies

Benzoic acid

Sensitive type

A plump, apparently healthy person, who is prone to attacks of rheumatism and gout at times, and has liver and kidney problems.

Blatta orientalis

Blatta orientalis in brief

Remedy for serious asthma and allergies

Source of the remedy

The whole cockroach

Suggested uses

1. Asthma with lots of secretions, accumulation of phlegm that is difficult to cough up

2. Chronic bronchitis

3. Allergy

Site of action

• The respiratory system

• The immune system

Related remedies

Ipecac

Borax

Borax in brief

Remedy for mouth ulcers and hypersensitive skin rashes

Source of the remedy

Sodium borate

Main actions

Exquisitely tender mouth ulcers on the tongue and inside the cheek

Skin rashes, with blisters that suppurate very easily

Hypersensitivity and irritability

Fear of any movement involving leaning forward or going downwards (staircase, lift)

Suggested uses

1. Mouth ulcer, especially in infants

2. Genital herpes

Site of action
• The skin and membranes

Related remedies

Mercurius corrosivus

Bothrops

Source of the remedy
The venom of the yellow viper

Main actions
Increased clotting of the blood leading to thrombosis (blood clots)

Suggested uses
Wherever there is risk of blood clotting: in the veins or after a heart attack

Site of action
• The blood

• The blood vessels

Related remedies

Vipera, Lachesis, and Naja

Bovista

Source of the remedy
The whole fungus known as the 'Giant Puffball' is used while it is still fresh.

Main actions
Sensations of swelling, with visible swelling on the head and limbs, especially on waking. Heavy periods

Secondary signs
Eczema and urticaria with pronounced swelling

Modalities
Worse throughout the morning and during the night

Suggested uses
1. Periods that are very heavy, particularly at night

2. Pre-menstrual syndrome (swelling and weight gain in the week before a period)

3. Headaches, with the sensation that the skull is getting bigger

4. Stammering in children

Site of action
• The female reproductive system

• The central nervous system

Related remedies

Thuja, Apis mellifica and Ammonium carbonicum

Bromium

Source of the remedy
Bromine

Main actions
Violent, allergic chest complaints; laryngitis; hardening and swelling of the glands; asthma; acne

Modalities
• Aggravated by hot weather and cool nights

• Improved at sea and by the seaside

Site of action
• The respiratory system

• The lymphatic and immune systems

Bromium

Kali bromatum, Coralium rubrum, Badiaga, Spongia tosta, Hepar sulphur and Medorrhinum

Bryonia alba

Bryonia alba in brief

• Major remedy (polychrest)

• For dryness in the membranes

• Swellings and fluid collections in the body cavities

• Influenza

• Constipation

Source of the remedy
The root of the White Bryony plant

Main actions
Dryness in the membranes, particularly in the respiratory and digestive systems; drying up of the secretions in these systems, resulting in great thirst; fluid in the lining of the lung, heart, abdomen, and joints, with effects on the affected organs

Secondary signs
Acute, piercing pains that become agonizing when touched. Aggravated by the slightest movement, heat in any form, being touched, after meals, on waking up, around 9 p.m. and by anger. Improved by rest, immobility, cold drinks, and lying on the painful side

Suggested uses
1. Acute or chronic inflammations, with or without fever, that appear in cold, damp weather: pleurisy, pneumonia, acute arthritis, tracheitis, and bronchitis with a dry cough, acute breast pain

2. Fever that comes on gradually in an exhausted, immobile subject, with intense thirst, sour sweat that provides relief, and headaches aggravated by movement

3. Upset stomach, acute inflammation of the gall bladder, and chronic constipation

Site of action
• The general condition during infection (influenza)

• The lining of the lungs, heart, abdomen, and joints

• The joints

• The intestinal tract

Rhus toxicodendron and Apis mellifica

This is often a swarthy, robust, muscular subject, a big eater who is afraid of heat and who is quick-tempered

Bufo rana

Bufo rana in brief
Minor remedy for mental retardation in children

Source of the remedy
The venomous liquid contained in the glands on the sides of the toad's back

Main actions
Localized inflammation with burning pains and skin infections; spasms and cramps followed by convulsions; sexual excitement followed by confusion and exhaustion

Secondary signs
Retarded development

Modalities
Aggravated by heat and noise; improved in a cool place

Suggested uses
1. Mental retardation

2. Whitlows

3. Frequent masturbation

Site of action
• The central nervous system

• The emotional state

Cactus grandiflorus

Cactus grandiflorus in brief
Remedy for the coronary arteries

Source of the remedy
Young stems of the Night-Blooming Cereus plant, found in Mexico

Main actions
Tight, constrictive feeling, like a vice around the heart

Suggested uses
1. Angina

2. Over-tired sportsmen with tired hearts

3. In smokers

Site of action
The heart.

Related remedies

Cuprum metallicum

Cadmium sulphuricum
Origin of the remedy
Cadmium Sulphate

Main actions
Stomach ulcers and cancers with a deterioration of general health. Deterioration of general health with increased fatigue and exhaustion

Suggested uses
1. As a preventive measure in subjects exposed to radiation

2. In exhausted alcoholics

3. Gastro-enteritis with bleeding

4. Facial paralysis after a cold snap

Site of action
• The general health

• The digestive system

Related remedies

X-Ray, Radium bromatum, Arsenicum album, Phosphorus, and Aconite

Cajuputum
Source of the remedy
Cajuput Oil

Main actions
Spasms in the larynx and the digestive

Homeopathy encyclopedia

tract; acid reflux from the stomach, with laryngeal irritation and cough

Site of action
- The larynx

- The stomach

Related remedies

Nux vomica and Robinia

Caladium
Caladium in brief
Remedy for impotence

Source of the remedy
The whole of the plant American Arum

Main actions
Impotence with increased sexual desire; nervous weakness; depression

Secondary signs
Smoking despite an intolerance to tobacco; memory loss

Suggested uses
Impotence with sexual excitation

Site of action
Male sexual organs

Related remedies

Agnus castus

Calcarea carbonica

Calcarea fluorica in brief
- Major remedy (polycrest)

- For recurrent ear, nose, and throat infections (children and adults)

- Children's growth and development

- Eczema in children

- Obesity in adults

- Depression in adults

Source of the remedy
The middle third of the Oyster Shell

Main actions
Deformations and bony protuberances; swelling of the neck glands; tendency to congestion; hypertension (high blood pressure); polyps in the nose, vagina, and bladder; sensitivity to the cold

Secondary signs
Excretions with sour and acid smell; craving for indigestible food; craving for eggs, ice creams, and sweet things; aversion to meat; intense craving for, or aversion to, milk, which is badly tolerated.

Modalities
- Aggravated by all forms of cold, by physical and intellectual exertion, a full moon, damp

- Improved by dry weather and when constipated

Suggested uses
1. In children: infections of the nose and pharynx, tonsillitis, ear infection, repeated bronchitis. Eczema in infants. Developmental delay (delay in walking). Digestive disorders

2. In adults: obesity, gout, pre-diabetes. Gallstones or stones in the urinary tract. Some types of high blood pres-

sure. Eczema, migraines, osteoarthritis. Polyps

Site of action
• General metabolism in an obese subject

• Development in a child

• The emotional state in anxious or sensitive subjects

• The immune system

Related remedies

Sulphur

Sensitive type

Rather small, stocky people with short arms, a solid bone structure, and powerful muscles, with a tendency to be overweight; these people give the impression of calm physical strength.

They have a stable, realistic personality and obey the law. They are slow, but precise and methodical, patient and persevering, cautious in their judgements, inclined to rationalize, sociable, and conservative. They are well organized, sometimes to the point of obsession, and will feel at home in any situation where little personal initiative is required. They make excellent civil servants or soldiers, sticking to all the regulations. Their lack of emotional display and introverted nature makes them passive.

They hate any surprises and so plan their lives. They mistrust and avoid any-thing abstract or surreal, science fiction, or the esoteric.

Calcarea fluorica

Calcarea fluorica in brief
• Growing problems

• Excessive laxity of the joints

• Varicose veins and related eczema

Source of the remedy
Calcium Fluoride

Main actions
Disorders of bone nutrition; hard, swollen lymph glands; lax tissues, double joints, prolapse, varicose veins, and hernia; chapped areas of hard skin, tending to infection.

Modalities
• Aggravated by movement and by cold, wet weather

• Improved by heat and by excessive movement

Suggested uses
1. Growth disorders (curved spine/scoliosis). Instability and backwardness in school
2. Repeated sprains. Prolapse of organs
3. Varicose veins and related eczema
4. Hard, swollen lymph glands. Benign lumps in the breasts, ovaries, or uterus

Site of action
• The immune system

• The skeletal system

• The veins

Homeopathy encyclopedia

Related remedies

Silica

Sensitive type

These people are of small or average size and often have deformed bones, lax ligaments, irregular teeth, and a tendency to sprains and prolapse.

Calcarea phosphorica

Calcarea phosphorica in brief
• Remedy for bone growth disorders

• Healing fractures

Source of the remedy
Calcium Phosphate

Main actions
Weight loss; disorders of the growth of bones, delayed healing of fractures, rickets; teething problems; fatigue; anaemia, and lymphatic problems

Secondary signs
Pains in the tips of bones; vaginal discharge; strong craving for ham, smoked meats, and lard

Modalities
• Aggravated by damp cold, consolation, or comforting, and thinking about the illness

• Improved in summer and by hot, dry weather

Suggested uses
1. Children: rickets, weight loss, problems with teething, a tendency to chronic infections in the nose and pharynx with swollen glands

2. Pain at the growth plates of bones in adolescence, acne, and headaches

3. Adult: healing fractures

Site of action
• The bones and joints

• The general health

Related remedies

Kali phosphoricum, Calcarea carbonica, and Calcarea fluorica.

Sensitive type

The constitutional Calcarea phosphorica is tall and thin, with long but straight bones. He, or she, is quickly tired by intellectual work, but is intelligent and often enthusiastic. There is little taste for steady work in view of the nervous and restless nature.

Calcarea picrata
Source of the remedy
Calcium Picrate

Suggested uses
Minor remedy for eczema in the ear canal

Calcarea sulphurica
Source of the remedy
Calcium Sulphate

Main actions
Painless chronic infections, especially of the skin: impetigo, acne. Chronic

lung infections with copious amounts of phlegm and no fever

Site of action
The immune system

Related remedies

Pulsatilla, Kali sulphuricum, and Silica

Calendula officinalis

Source of the remedy
The fresh leaves and flowers of the Marigold

Suggested uses
This remedy is particularly used externally as diluted mother tincture, or in the form of an ointment or cream; it is the homeopaths' antiseptic and healing substance. In internal use, at low potencies, such as 6C, it has an analgesic and antiseptic action on lacerated and infected wounds.

Camphora

Source of the remedy
Natural camphor obtained from the gum of the camphor tree

Main actions
Common cold that appears very suddenly; sudden feeling of intense cold; fainting with cardiovascular failure; drop in blood pressure with loss of consciousness

Modalities
Aggravated by the cold

Site of action
The immune system

Cantharis vesicatoria

Cantharis in brief
• Remedy for acute cystitis

• Effusion in the serous membranes

• Skin burns

Source of the remedy
The beetle known as the Spanish Fly used whole

Main actions
Acute inflammations with intense burning in the urinary system and genitals; pains before, during, and after passing urine; fluid collections in the lungs, abdomen, brain and joints; blisters on the skin, with intense burning pains

Secondary signs
Very violent, smarting, burning pains in the region of the kidneys, spreading to the bladder; general stinging pains and intense burning sensations

Modalities
• Aggravated when passing urine and by touch

• Improved by heat and hot applications

Suggested uses
1. Acute cystitis. Kidney infections. Urine retention

2. Partial thickness skin burns. All burning rashes

3. All fluid collections in the organs, with burning pains improved by heat

4. Certain types of eczema

Homeopathy encyclopedia

Site of action
- The bladder and the urinary system

- The skin

Related remedies

Bryonia alba, Borax, Staphysagria, and Apis mellifica

Capsicum

Capsicum in brief
Remedy for ear infections

Source of the remedy
Dried Cayenne Pepper

Main actions
Irritation and inflammation with intense burning (similar to that caused by pepper) in the digestive, respiratory, and urinary systems. Painful ear infections

Secondary signs
Great sensitivity to cold; thirst for cold water

Modalities
- Aggravated by cold and contact

- Improved by heat

Suggested uses
1. Ear infections especially at the start

2. Infections in the nose and pharynx with a burning sensation, as if caused by pepper

Site of action
The ear, nose, and throat

Related remedies

Ferrum Phosphoricum and Apis mellifica.

Carbo animalis

Source of the remedy
Animal Charcoal

Main actions
Poor circulation in the hands, feet, and face, with blue discoloration; varicose veins and varicose ulcers; poor general health; cancer; hard, swollen glands; ulcers

Modalities
Aggravated by the cold

Suggested uses
1. Circulatory problems in the face and limbs

2. Varicose veins and ulcers

3. Acne rosacea

4. All chronic diseases with poor general health

Site of action
- The veins

- The general health

- The immune system

Related remedies

Calcarea fluorica, Lachesis, and Lueticum

Carbo vegetabilis

Carbo vegetabilis in brief
- Remedy for faintness in elderly subjects

- Flatulence

Source of the remedy
Vegetable Charcoal

Main actions
Flatulence. Progressive problems of the circulation, with varicose veins and ulcers. Progressive loss of strength with general weakness, prostration, and a tendency to heart problems. Heaviness in the chest

Secondary signs
The entire body is cold but the person feels as if he or she is burning inside. Irritating, foul-smelling discharges. Aversion to fatty foods, meat, and milk

Modalities
• Aggravated by fatty foods and dairy products, in the evening, in winter, by humid heat, by wine

• Improved by cold, by being fanned

Suggested uses
1. Serious conditions in elderly people: chronic weakness and weight loss, asthma, and heart failure

2. Whooping cough in a weak child

3. Flatulence and wind

4. Certain types of varicose ulcers

Site of action
• The general health

• The immune system

Related remedies

China, Thuja, and Antimonium tartaricum

Sensitive type

They are tired, weak, elderly people with poor digestion and swelling above the navel. They are intolerant to alcohol, are sensitive to cold, and need fresh air.

Carbolic acid
Source of the remedy
Phenol

Main actions
Blisters and ulcers on the skin and membranes, which are prone to infection. Eczema on the hands with itching. Generalized eczema affecting the general health. Serious infections with weakness (treatment in combination with antibiotics)

Site of action
• The immune system

• The skin

Related remedies

Cantharis, Pyrogen, and Arsenicum album

Carboneum sulphuratum
Source of the remedy
Carbon Bisulphide

Main actions
Reduced sensory perception; reduced hearing; reduced sharpness of vision; problems with keeping balance; lapses of memory. Polyneuritis (inflammation of the nerves). All neurological diseases and alcoholic polyneuritis (inflamma-

tion of the nerves). Anaemia with pallor and sensitivity to cold

Site of action
• The general health

• The immune system

Related remedies

Ether, Sulphuric acid and Argentum nitricum

Carduus marianus
Carduus marianus in brief
Remedy for drainage of the liver

Source of the remedy
The seeds of the Milk Thistle plant

Main actions
Congestion and swelling of the liver

Suggested uses
'Drainage' remedy that improves the functioning of the liver when it is stressed. It is used as a complement to the major constitutional remedies.

Site of action
The liver and gall bladder

Related remedies

Berberis vulgaris and Lycopodium

Castor equi
Source of the remedy
The thumbnail of the Horse

Suggested uses
This remedy is used as an ointment to prevent cracks from appearing in the nipples during breast-feeding; one application after each feed

Castoreum
Source of the remedy
Secretions from the foreskin of the male beaver

Main actions
Excessive sexual excitability in men; hysteria; spasms in the respiratory and digestive systems; spasms of the large bowel

Site of action
• The male reproductive system

• The central nervous system and the nerves

Related remedies

Moschus, Ambra grisea, and Ignatia

Caulophyllum
Caulophyllum in brief
Major remedy given to women preparing to give birth and for period problems

Source of the remedy
The root of the Blue Cohosh plant

Main actions
• Spasms of pain in the pelvis and period problems

• Intermittent pains in the small joints

Suggested uses
1. Preparation for giving birth

2. Pain on the first day of the periods, which tends to be light

3. Pains in the small joints, when these pains often move from site to site

Site of action
- The female reproductive system

- The small joints

Related remedies

Cimicifuga and Colocynthis

Causticum
Causticum in brief
- Constipation

- Urine retention

- Hoarseness, dry cough

- Warts under the nails

- Scars from burns

Source of the remedy
Distillation of a mixture of recently slaked lime and potassium sulphate

Main actions
Severe weakness, depression, and increased sensitivity; slow and progressive paralysis of the face, larynx, and sphincters (muscles in the orifices); scar tissues; contractures and stiffness; warts

Secondary signs
Constipation with desire to open the bowels; urinary retention with incomplete emptying of the bladder; urinary incontinence; hoarseness worse in the morning, improved by a mouthful of cold water; dry cough with a feeling that there is a wound in the windpipe; warts under the nails; burning pains; craving for smoked and spicy food; aversion to sweet things; complaints mainly found on the right side of the body

Modalities
Aggravated by cold, dry weather and thinking about the illness; improved by hot, humid weather and by drinking a mouthful of cold water

Suggested uses
1. Constipation

2. Paralysis of the bladder with urine retention and inability to void. Urinary incontinence while coughing, sneezing, or laughing, or while asleep

3. Hoarseness as described above

4. Dry cough as described above

5. Warts under the nails

6 Scars caused by old burns. Troublesome scars from burns

Site of action
- The bowels and the bladder

- The respiratory system

- The skin

Related remedies

Aconite, Sepia, Graphites, Arnica, and Cuprum metallicum

Sensitive type

A thin, elderly person who is sad and cries over nothing.

Ceanothus americana
Source of the remedy
The leaves of the Californian lilac

Suggested uses
Pains on the left side of the abdomen

coming from the spleen, especially in malaria. This remedy is very rarely used.

Cedron

Source of the remedy
The dried seed of a small American tree, the Rattlesnake Bean

Main actions
Headaches, neuralgia, or fevers that recur hourly

Modalities
Aggravation in a hot, humid climate and always at exactly the same time

Suggested uses
1. Neuralgia, headaches, or migraines that recur at precisely the same time

2. Malaria.

3. Epilepsy recurring in every menstrual cycle

Site of action
The central nervous system

Related remedies

Aranea diadema, Arsenicum album, Natrum muriaticum and China

Chamomilla

Chamomilla in brief
• Teething problems in children

• Behavioural problems in children

• Emotionally disturbed adults

Source of the remedy
The entire German Camomile plant, in bloom

Main actions
Hypersensitivity to pain; digestive problems; emotional disturbances: the person becomes irritable, capricious, behaves badly, and is always discontented.

Secondary signs
Sleepy in the day, insomnia at night; intolerable pains with numbness; restlessness

Modalities
• Aggravated by anger, heat (in the case of toothaches), from 9p.m. to midnight, when reprimanded, during teething, and by coffee

• Improvement when held in the arms (in children) or when travelling in a car

Suggested uses
1. Teething problems in a well-behaved infant who becomes bad-tempered and unbearable, sometimes with fever, diarrhoea, and mild bronchitis

2. Behavioural problems in hypersensitive, bad-tempered, and discontented people

3. Intolerable pain, whatever the cause, if the characteristics and modalities of the medicine are present

Site of action
• The nervous system: pain

• Psychological: behavioural problems

Related remedies

Nux vomica

Sensitive type

This remedy, often thought to be only for children, is perfectly suitable for those unbearable, demanding, spiteful, dependent, and highly sensitive people who continually accuse everyone of treating them badly. They are prone to extremely violent angry outbursts. These highly immature people are incapable of taking on responsibility. They are maladjusted, very impressionable, and driven to distraction by the least pain. Their temper fits can cause digestive problems (stomach cramps, abdominal swelling, or diarrhoea) cardiovascular disorders (palpitations, heavy sensation in the chest), or, in women, disrupted menstrual cycles. There is no particular body type; the only physical characteristic is a stomach frequently bloated, due to wind.

Chelidonium majus

Chelidonium majus in brief
A 'drainage remedy' for the liver

Source of the remedy
The Greater Celandine herb, whole and in bloom

Main actions
Painful swelling of the liver; pain spreading to the tip of the right shoulder blade; breath with a foul smell; sleepiness after meals

Secondary signs
Right-sided remedy; stools, urine, tongue, and vaginal discharge all a golden-yellow colour; aversion to cheese

Modalities
Aggravated by movement, at 4 a.m. and 4 p.m. Improved by resting, by eating, or drinking something hot

Suggested uses
Disorders of the liver and digestion

Site of action
The liver

Related remedies

Berberis, Carduus marianus, and Lycopodium

Sensitive type

The remedy acts particularly well on Lycopodium-type subjects.

Chenopodium
Source of the remedy
The Jerusalem Oak, whole and in bloom

Main actions
Progressive deafness; abnormal noises in the ear; vertigo with deafness; Ménière's syndrome

Site of action
The ear

Related remedies

China, Phosphorus, and Lycopodium

Chimaphila
Source of the remedy
The Ground Holly plant, used whole

Chimaphila

Main actions
Difficulties in passing urine; urinary tract infection with pus in the urine; enlargement of the prostate

Site of action
The urinary and reproductive systems, particularly in men

Related remedies

Sabal serulata, Conium and Thuja

China officinalis
China in brief
• Remedy with a general action

• For prolonged fever

• Intermittent fever

• The after-effects of a sickness in which there has been fluid loss

Source of the remedy
Cinchona, the bark of a tree that grows in the Andes. It was the first remedy with which Hahnemann experimented, leading to the development of homeopathy.

Main actions
The physical and emotional strength is sapped, just as in prolonged fevers or after loss of body fluids (haemorrhages, sweating, diarrhoea, vomiting, and prolonged breast-feeding).

Low blood pressure with dizziness, headaches, and weakness of the heart

Secondary signs
Hypersensitivity to being touched

(especially on the scalp); throbbing headaches; ringing in the ear; the problems appear every other day

Modalities
• Aggravated by the slightest contact, through loss of body fluid (haemorrhages, sweating, and diarrhoea) and by draughts

• Improved by heat and by firm pressure

Suggested uses
1. Haemorrhages and diarrhoea

2. Convalescence after fevers and haemorrhages

Site of action
• The general health

• The circulation

• Fluid balance

Related remedies

Belladonna, Millefolium, Kali phosphoricum, and Carbo vegetabilis

Sensitive type

All debilitated and weak people. It is rare for energetic people to need China.

China sulphuricum
Source of the remedy
Quinine Sulphate

Main actions
Vertigo, abnormal noises in the ear, deafness (although the remedy only has a very limited efficacy in such

cases). Pain from disease of the spine in the neck and upper chest. Headaches and neuralgia

Site of action
The ear and the spinal column

Related remedies

China and Cimicifuga

Chionothus virginica
Source of the remedy
The bark from the root of the Fringe tree

Main actions
Enlargement of the liver with jaundice, nausea, and colourless stools. Gallstones; spasms of pain in the region of the gall bladder; headaches and migraines with liver disorders

Site of action
The liver and gall bladder

Related remedies

Carduus marianus, Bryonia, Chelidonium, Chenopodium, Berberis, and Hydrastis

Cholesterinum
Source of the remedy
Crystals of Cholesterol

Main actions
High cholesterol levels; slow digestion; constipation; high blood pressure; gallstones

Suggested uses
1. This remedy does not reduce the levels of cholesterol in the blood

2. Gallstones, if they are made of cholesterol

3. Yellowish deposits of cholesterol under the skin (especially around the eyelids)

Site of action
The metabolism of fats

Related remedies

Lycopodium and Phosphorus

Cicuta virosa
Source of the remedy
The root of the Fool's Parsley plant

Main actions
Spasms, convulsions

Generalized epilepsy (grand mal) and localized fits (petit mal); tetanus; eruption of blisters and pustules on the skin

Modalities
Aggravated by touch, light, noise, and the cold

Suggested uses
1. All muscle spasms

2. Epilepsy in conjunction with the classical treatments. A professional homeopath must treat the patient

Site of action
The central nervous system

Related remedies

Sulphur, Arsenicum album, Psorinum and Stramonium

Cimex

Source of the remedy
The Common Bedbug

Main actions
Stiffness and contractions in the ligaments and muscles of the legs, following exercise; inflammation of the nose; colds with pains in the sinuses in the forehead

Site of action
• The nerves

• The ear, nose, and throat

Related remedies

Arnica and Cuprum metallicum

Cimicifuga

Cimicifuga in brief
• Problems with periods, pregnancy, and childbirth

• Problems with the joints

Source of the remedy
The roots of the Black Cohosh plant, also known as Actea racemosa

Main actions
Highly excitable nerves and muscles, especially in women, with spasms and pains in the pelvis; excitation of the central nervous system

Secondary signs
Period problems with pains proportional to the intensity of the blood flow; irregular periods; searing, cramp-like pains with twitching of the muscles; pain in the Achilles tendon

Modalities
• Aggravated by the damp cold, during periods according to the heaviness of the flow

• Improved by the open air, eating, and heat

Suggested uses
1. All period problems where the symptoms are directly related to the rate of flow

2. Emotional problems in pregnancy

3. Cramp-like rheumatic pains and tendonitis

4. The control of labour before delivery

Site of action
• The female reproductive system

• The joints

Sensitive type

A woman who talks constantly and incoherently. Sadness and hopelessness alternate with periods of excitement. The emotional problems often alternate with physical disorders (rheumatism).

Cina

Cina in brief
Remedy for nervous irritability in children

Source of the remedy
The unexploded seed heads of the Wormseed plant

Main actions
Convulsions in one half of the body, with breathing difficulties and urinary

incontinence; problems in distinguishing colours; appearance of a squint; worm infestations

Secondary signs
Anal and nasal itching; constant, insatiable hunger; gnawing, piercing pains around the navel; restless sleep with night terrors

Modalities
• Aggravated by the new moon and by being touched

• Improved by lying on the stomach

Suggested uses
1. Nervous irritability in children with worms. Behavioural disorders

2. Bed-wetting

3. Cramping abdominal pains

4. Spasmodic cough

Site of action
The central nervous system

Related remedies

Stramonium and Hyoscyamus

Sensitive type

Unpleasant, whining, stubborn, demanding, and perpetually dissatisfied children. They hate being touched or looked at. They often have bluish shadows under the eyes. They yawn frequently, grind their teeth at night, and sleep restlessly.

Cinnabaris
Source of the remedy
Mercuric sulphide, or Cinnabar

Main actions
Bright red rash on the face and genitals; frontal sinusitis with burning pains; post-nasal catarrh; warts that bleed easily

Site of action
• The skin

• The ear, nose, and throat

• The genitals

Related remedies

Lueticum, Aurum metallicum, Capsicum, Kali bichromicum, Nitric acid, and Thuja

Cistus canadensis
Source of the remedy
The Rock Rose, used whole

Suggested uses
1. Chronic enlargement and hardening of the nodes

2. Extreme sensitivity to cold

3. Intolerance of the cold, with a feeling of localized chilliness

Modalities
• Aggravated by cold

• Better for eating

Site of action
The immune system

Related remedies

Silica and Calcarea Carbonica

Homeopathy encyclopedia

Clemetis erecta

Source of the remedy
The young leafy stems of the Clematis Erecta plant, when it starts to flower

Suggested uses
1. Inflammations and infections of the urethra (urethritis) and the testicles (orchitis)

2. Vaginal discharge

3. Eczema, with blistering, all over the scalp

4. This remedy is used by homeopaths, in conjunction with antibiotic treatment

Site of action
• The urinary and reproductive systems

• The skin

Related remedies

Thuja, Medorrhinum, Cantharis, and Mercurius vivus.

Coca

Source of the remedy
The leaf of the Coca shrub, used by the Incas, contains cocaine

Main actions
Insomnia at high altitudes with headaches, anxiety, and respiratory disorders. Mountain sickness

Site of action
• The central nervous system

• The cardiovascular system

Related remedies

Arsenicum album

Cocculus indicus

Cocculus indicus in brief
Remedy for travel sickness

Source of the remedy
The seeds of the tree known as Indian Cockle

Main actions
Nausea, vomiting, and dizziness; paralytic weakness (knees giving way); period problems, in women, with great weakness, nausea, and dizziness

Secondary signs
Nausea and dizziness with great lethargy, especially in cars, boats, or trains. Aversion to all food. Craving for cold drinks

Modalities
• Aggravated at night and by insomnia, passive movements (car, train, boat), tobacco smoke

• Improved by heat

Suggested uses
1. Travel sickness, especially if improved by heat

2. Insomnia after overworking

3. Morning sickness

4. Period problems with great weakness, nausea, and vertigo

5. Nausea and dizziness in general

Collinsonia canadensis

Site of action
The central nervous system

Related remedies

Tabacum

Coccus cacti

Source of the remedy
The Cochineal is an insect that infests cacti. The remedy is prepared from the dried bodies of the females.

Main actions
Coughing fits with thick phlegm; thick, runny discharge from the nose; whooping cough; heavy periods with black blood

Modalities
• Aggravated in the morning and by the heat of a bed

• Improved by cold drinks

Site of action
• The respiratory system

• The blood

• The female reproductive system

Related remedies

Drosera, Hydrastis, and Corallium rubrum

Coffea cruda

Source of the remedy
The Coffee Bean, before roasting

Main actions
Insomnia, feeling of euphoria, heightened senses. Increased mental activity with a torrent of ideas, leading to insomnia. Overactive thyroid glands in coffee drinkers

Modalities
Aggravated by coffee and all stimulants, by noise, and by joyful emotions

Site of action
The central nervous system

Related remedies

China, Chamomilla, Lachesis, and Ignatia

Colchicum autumnale

Colchicum autumnale in brief
Remedy for gout

Source of the remedy
The bulb of the Autumn Crocus, gathered at the beginning of summer

Main actions
Weakness; severe diarrhoea with a great deal of wind; pains that quickly move from one joint to another; acute pain in the big toe, which is very tender to the touch

Suggested uses
Rheumatism in subjects prone to gout

Collinsonia canadensis

Source of the remedy
The dry root of the Stone-Root plant

Main actions
Very painful haemorrhoids, especially in pregnancy; constipation with haemorrhoids that bleed easily

Site of action
The veins

Aesculus, Hamamelis, and Arnica

Colocynthis

Colocynthis in brief
- Remedy for gall bladder and digestive spasms

- Neuralgia

Source of the remedy
The fruit of the Bitter Cucumber plant

Main actions
Intense irritation of the digestive system; violent nervous irritation with spasms in the stomach, gall bladder, bowel, and bladder; severe neuralgia in the face and sciatica

Secondary signs
Violent spasms of pain

Modalities
Aggravated by anger and indignation; improved by bending over double, by strong pressure, heat, and movement

Suggested uses
1. Painful diarrhoea, colic, and gall bladder colic

2. Kidney colic (especially on the left-hand side)

3. Period problems

4. Facial neuralgia (especially on the left)

5. Sciatica (especially on the left)

Site of action
- The digestive system

- The liver and gall bladder

- The urinary system

- The nervous system

Related remedies

Magnesia phosphorica

Sensitive type

Corpulent, irritable, quick-tempered subject who easily becomes ill

Conium maculatum

Conium maculatum in brief
Remedy for dizziness, paralysis, hard, swollen glands, and impotence

Source of the remedy
The whole Poison Hemlock, in flower

Main actions
Visual problems; dizziness; paralysis; hard, swollen glands, breasts, and testicles

Secondary signs
Impotence with intense sexual desire; abundant sweating on going to sleep; intense craving for salt with great thirst; intense watering of the eye, with fear of the light; aversion to milk and bread

Modalities
- Aggravated by celibacy, the cold, the night, alcohol, artificial light, and when lying down (in the case of dizzy spells)

- Improved by heat

Suggested uses

1. Dizziness
2. Impotence due to celibacy
3. Nervous weakness, after celibacy
4. Mastitis (painful, lumpy breasts)

Site of action

- The nervous system
- The glands

Related remedies

Argentum nitricum, Agnus castus, and Phytolacca

Sensitive type

This is often an elderly, tired, depressed person who does not like to be contradicted. However, the remedy often acts on dizzy spells, at any age.

Corallium rubrum

Source of the remedy
Red Coral

Main actions
Coughing fits like whooping cough. Inflammation of the nose, larynx, and pharynx, with spasms and thick phlegm

Modalities
Aggravated by contact with fresh air

Site of action

- The respiratory system
- The immune system

Related remedies

Coccus cacti and Drosera

Crataegus

Source of the remedy
The fresh berries of the Hawthorn

Suggested uses
Heart tonic, in cases of moderately raised blood pressure

Site of action
The cardiovascular system

Related remedies

Pulsatilla, Arsenicum iodatum, and Aurum metallicum

Crocus sativa

Source of the remedy
The dry stigmas of Saffron

Main actions
Heavy periods with black blood; changeable moods with obsessive fantasies

Site of action
The female reproductive system

Related remedies

Secale cornutum and Sabina

Crotalus horridus

Source of the remedy
Venom of the Brazilian rattlesnake

Main actions
Haemorrhages of black blood that will not clot

Site of action
The blood

Homeopathy encyclopedia

Phosphorus, Lachesis, and Hamamelis

Croton tiglium

Croton tiglium in brief
Remedy for eczema and herpes

Source of the remedy
The oil of the seeds of the Croton Tiglium plant

Main action
Skin irritation with itchy blisters; intestinal irritation with severe diarrhoea; alternating skin and gut symptoms

Secondary signs
The blisters rapidly become infected, leading to yellow scabs and outbreaks on another part of the body. Intense itching. Burning sensation on very delicate skin. Watery, yellow diarrhoea, expelled in a jet, after eating or drinking only a very small amount

Modalities
Aggravated by touch and the slightest intake of food or drink, and in summer

Suggested uses
1. Eczema

2. Herpes on the face

3. Eye inflammations

4. Diarrhoea after taking antibiotics

Site of action
• The skin

• The intestines

Rhus toxicodendron

Cuprum metallicum

Cuprum metallicum in brief
Remedy for cramps and spasms

Source of the remedy
The metal Copper

Main actions
Spasms and cramps in all the muscles, at varying sites and of varying intensity. Onset of gastro-enteritis

Secondary signs
Regular recurrence of symptoms; violent cramps in the calves and feet; violent convulsions; dry, spasmodic cough, similar to whooping cough; very violent stomach cramps with nausea and vomiting; hiccups

Modalities
Aggravated at night, touch, pressure, and on a new moon. Improved by drinking cold water

Suggested uses
1. Cramps in general

2. Spasms in the digestive and respiratory systems

3. Convulsions and muscle spasms

Site of action
The nervous system and muscles

Zincum metallicum

Sensitive type

These sensitive individuals have a highly changeable personality and lose their temper easily. However, this remedy acts on all cramps and spasms, regardless of the personality and age.

Cyclamen europaeum

Cyclamen europaeum in brief
Remedy for migraines with visual disturbance

Source of the remedy
The tuber from the plant of the same name

Main actions
Headaches, vertigo with visual disturbance: objects seem to move. Irregular periods with black blood with many clots, with pain before and during the period

Secondary signs
Very marked aversion to coffee, but also to fat, butter, and meat

Modalities
• Aggravated by the open air, by coffee, by fat

• Improved by heat, by the arrival of periods, by movement

Suggested uses
1. Migraines during periods

2. Migraines with visual disturbances

3. Period problems

Site of action
• The blood vessels

• The central nervous system

Related remedies

Tuberculinum koch

Dioscorea villosa

Source of the remedy
The dry root of the Wild Yam, collected in autumn

Main actions
Pain, which comes in spasms, in the stomach, intestine, and uterus; neuralgia, improved by bending backwards; colic in infants; sciatic pains

Site of action
The nerves

Related remedies

Helonias, Trillium pendulum and Bryonia alba

Diptherinum (Diptheria nosode)

Source of the remedy
A nosode prepared from Diphtheria bacteria or from the membrane caused by the infection

Suggested uses
Recurrent tonsillitis, laryngitis with a feeling of suffocation

Site of action
The immune system

Related remedies

Streptococcinum, Hepar sulphur, Silica and Tuberculinum

Dolichos pruriens

Source of the remedy
The whole pod of the plant popularly known as 'Cow-itch'

Suggested uses
Itching, with or without a rash; itching in elderly people; itching with jaundice

Modalities
Aggravated at night, by the heat of the bed.

Site of action
• The skin

• The liver

Related remedies

Psorinum, Sulphur, and Urtica Urens

Drosera rotundifolia

Source of the remedy
The Round-Leaved Sundew used whole

Suggested uses
• Troublesome cough as with whooping cough

• Laryngitis with a troublesome cough, vomiting, and runny discharges

• Inflamed glands

• General poor health

Modalities
Aggravated after midnight, when going to bed, and by heat

Site of action
• The respiratory system

• The immune system

Related remedies

Cuprum metallicum, Baryta iodata and Coccus cacti

Dulcamara

Dulcamara in brief
Major remedy for all conditions aggravated by cold, damp weather

Source of the remedy
The young leafy, flowering stem of the Woody Nightshade

Main actions
Intense sensitivity to damp cold weather, leading to symptoms of a cold, diarrhoea, swelling of the glands, and rheumatic pains. Warts on the skin and moist, itchy rashes

Secondary signs
General sensitivity to the cold and damp; feeling of being bruised; rashes alternating with rheumatism and diarrhoea

Modalities
• Aggravated by damp, cold, or rainy weather, at night, and at rest

• Improved by heat and dry weather and by movement

Suggested uses

1. All respiratory, digestive, and joint complaints following exposure to damp cold (diarrhoea, dry or loose cough, swollen glands, rheumatism)

2. Flat warts on the back of the hand

Site of action

- The respiratory system

- The skeletal system

- The digestive system

- The skin

Related remedies

Rhus toxicodendron, Ruta, Thuja and Bryonia

Sensitive type

A fat person with cellulite, very sensitive to damp cold

Echinacea angustifolia

Source of the remedy
The whole Echinacea plant, also known as the Purple Cone-Flower

Main actions
Abscesses, septic conditions, infections with pus, and infected lymph glands. Remedy for infections and blood poisoning, used in conjunction with antibiotics

Site of action
The immune system

Related remedies

Pyrogen, Hepar sulph, and Silica

Eel serum

See Serum anguillae

Equisetum hyemale

Source of the remedy
The fresh Horse-tail herb, picked in spring

Main actions
It acts on the urinary tract, especially the bladder

Secondary signs
Children who bed-wet frequently; urinary infections with pains in the bladder, that are not relieved by passing urine; feeling of heaviness in the abdomen and bladder; pain during and, especially, after passing urine

Modalities
Aggravated by movement and by pressure

Suggested uses
1. Bed-wetting in children

2. Acute or chronic urinary tract infection

Erigeron canadensis

Source of the remedy
The Fleabane plant, whole and in bloom

Main actions
Profuse haemorrhages of bright red blood: from the respiratory system, the urinary tract, and the nose, and heavy periods with spasms and pains

Modalities
Aggravated by the slightest movement.

Site of action
The blood

Related remedies

China, Phosphorus and Chamomilla

Eryngium aquaticum
Source of the remedy
The Button Snakeroot plant

Main actions
Irritation of the bladder and urethra; irritation of the larynx, leading to a continuous productive cough; sexual problems in men with poor sperm counts

Suggested uses
1. Pain in the urethra in men with prostate problems

2. Laryngitis with a constant burning feeling

3. Weak or absent erections with leakage of secretions from the prostate or ejaculate

Site of action
• The reproductive system

• The larynx

Related remedies

Agnus castus, Kali phosphoricum, and Mercurius vivus

Eugenia jambosa
Source of the remedy
The fresh seeds of the Rose-Apple plant

Suggested uses
Used in teenage acne and rosacea acne, especially in alcoholics

Eupatorium perfoliatum
Source of the remedy
The flowering top part of the Boneset plant

Suggested uses
• Remedy for influenza with violent aching and bone-breaking pains, fever, and soreness of the eyeballs

• Cough with chest pains

Site of action
The immune system

Related remedies

Gelsemium, Phytolacca, and Arnica

Euphorbium officinarum
Source of the remedy
The sap of the Euphorbium, a cactus-like plant; it is highly irritant

Main actions
Appearance of blisters with skin swelling; burning pains; eczema and shingles; all painful, inflammatory skin conditions with significant swelling

Site of action
• The skin

• The immune system

Related remedies

Cantharis, Mezereum, and Croton tiglium

Euphrasia

Source of the remedy
The herb Eyebright, used whole and in bloom

Main actions
Burning watery discharge from the eyes, and watery non-irritant nasal secretions, caused by hay fever or allergy. Non-infective conjunctivitis. All watery eye conditions

Modalities
Aggravated by the sun, the air, and the wind

Site of action
The eye

Related remedies
Allium cepa and Mixed pollens and grasses

Fagopyrum

Source of the remedy
The entire Buckwheat plant

Main actions
Itching, with or without skin rashes, especially in old age

Modalities
Aggravated by the heat and at the end of the afternoon

Site of action
The skin

Related remedies
Lycopodium and Dolichos

Ferrum metallicum

Source of the remedy
The metal Iron

Main actions
General fatigue and depression in pale anaemic people, with flushed cheeks. Haemorrhages, headaches, and intolerance of noise. Painless but exhausting diarrhoea. Dizziness and congestive headaches. Early heavy periods, that lead to exhaustion

Modalities
• Aggravation from the cold, in the night (diarrhoea)

• Better for gentle motion

Site of action
The general health

Related remedies
China, Kali carbonicum, and Phosphorus

Ferrum phosphoricum

Ferrum phosphoricum in brief
• Remedy for infections with slight fever

• Childhood illnesses with rashes

Source of the remedy
Iron Phosphate

Main actions
Infections with slight fever

Congestion and localized haemorrhages

Secondary signs
Rapid pulse with normal blood pres-

Homeopathy encyclopedia

sure; nosebleeds; face reddens and pales alternately; soft skin; very painful, spasmodic dry cough. Yellow phlegm

Modalities
• Aggravated by touching, movement, in the early hours of the morning

• Improved by cold applications

Suggested uses
1. Frequently used remedy for the first stages of illnesses with a slight fever

2. Illnesses with rashes, ear infections, bronchitis, sore throats, feverish colds, the onset of influenza. Tendency to nosebleeds

Site of action
• The immune system

• The respiratory system

• The circulation

Related remedies

Capsicum, Bryonia alba, Belladonna and Phosphorus

Sensitive type

This remedy is effective at the start of any illness

Fluoric acid
Source of the remedy
Hydrofluoric Acid

Main actions
Varicose veins; destructive, ulcerating conditions affecting the skin, bones and soft tissues; bedsores

Secondary signs
Excessively lax ligaments

Modalities
• Aggravated by heat and standing up

• Improved by strenuous physical activity and cold

Suggested uses
1. Varicose veins, varicose ulcers, and eczema associated with varicose veins

2. Dental caries/dental decay

3. Bone infections

Site of action
• The veins

• The teeth

Related remedies

Lueticum, Silica, Mercurius solubilis, and Phosphorus

Folliculinum
Source of the remedy
The follicle of a Human Ovary

Main actions
Painful swelling of the breasts, headaches, migraines, neuralgia, and depression before a period

Suggested uses
An excellent remedy to regulate the menstrual cycle in general, particularly helpful for the pre-menstrual syndrome

Formica rufa
Source of the remedy
The crushed live Red Ant

Main actions
Pain when urinating; remedy used to treat recurrent cystitis; certain types of arthritis

Site of action
- The urinary system

- The immune system

- The skeletal system

Related remedies

Mercurius vivus and Cantharis

Fraxinus americana
Source of the remedy
The bark of the White Ash tree

Main actions
Uterus: large fibroids that bleed easily, with a dragging sensation in the lower abdomen

Related remedies

Aurum muriaticum natronatum and Thuja

Gambogia
Source of the remedy
The resinous gum of the Gamboge tree

Main actions
Profuse watery diarrhoea, which irritates the anus, and is expelled suddenly and forcibly. Pains around the navel and gurgling noises in the abdomen

Modalities
Worse in the evening and at night

Site of action
The intestine

Related remedies

Chamomilla, Sulphur, Crocus, and Croton tiglium

Gelsemium
Gelsemium in brief
- Remedy with a general action

- For influenza

- Nervous conditions

Source of the remedy
The root of the Yellow Jasmine

Main actions
Fever with loss of energy, progressive paralysis, particularly in the respiratory muscles, slowing of the heart rate, and drop in blood pressure. Inflammatory conditions of the respiratory and digestive systems

Secondary signs
Trembling; mental and physical weakness; absence of thirst in fever; aches; shivers down the back; facial flushing; severe headaches; sensation that the heart has stopped beating

Modalities
- Aggravated by emotions, bad news, heat (the sun), hot stuffy rooms, tobacco, and storms

- Improved by sweating, stimulants, fresh air, slow movement, and passing large amounts of urine

Homeopathy encyclopedia

Suggested uses

1. Infections with profound weakness, especially influenza. The person is prostrate and trembling. Aches and shivers in the back. He or she is not thirsty

2. Nervous conditions, particularly the anticipation of events

3. Congestive headaches

Site of action
- The central nervous system

- Nerves and muscles

Sensitive type

Typically, the Gelsemium person trembles with fear and is very emotional. Attacks of nerves lead to diarrhoea. He or she wants to be left alone, but fears solitude. However, the remedy can be prescribed for this type of illness regardless of character.

Glonoine

Glonoine in brief
Remedy for hot flushes and extremely high blood pressure

Source of the remedy
Nitro-glycerine or TNT

Main actions
Disorders of the circulation with sudden, violent congestion in the head, palpitations, and dilated blood vessels

Secondary signs
Sudden onset of the symptoms

Modalities
- Aggravated by all kinds of heat

- Improved by the open air

Suggested uses

1. Heart: sensation of blood surging to the heart and arteries of the neck. Palpitations

2. Elevation of the blood pressure

3. Sensation of blood rushing violently into the head with throbbing (hot flushes in the menopause)

Site of action
The cardiovascular system

Related remedies

Sanguinaria and Belladonna

Gnaphalium

Source of the remedy
The Sweet Scented Everlasting flower, whole and in bloom

Main actions
Sciatica with cramp-like pains; neuralgia in general, alternating with numbness; diarrhoea with cramp-like pains

Site of action
- The nerves

- The intestines

Related remedies

Colocynthis

Graphites

Graphites in brief
Remedy for eczema, warts, scars, constipation

Source of the remedy
The lead of the finest English drawing pencils, the mineral Carbon in an almost pure form

Main actions
Irritating, cracked eczema with a thick honey coloured discharge. Flatulence and constipation, with no desire for bowel movements. Occasional diarrhoea. Reduced ovarian function. Reduced sexual drive in men. Thyroid insufficiency. Anaemia, swelling of the legs, and poor circulation. Hot flushes

Secondary signs
The person is sensitive to the cold

Modalities
• Aggravated by the cold, during and after periods

• Improved by wrapping up warm, by being in the open air, despite chilliness

Suggested uses
1. Eczema or impetigo, with dry skin and blisters containing thick, yellow fluid that resembles honey. The lesions bleed easily and are often located behind the ears, in the skin creases of the arms and legs, on the eyelids, the scalp, and the genital organs. They are itchy, burning, and aggravated by heat

2. Warts around the nails and cysts on the scalp

3. Thickened, hardened scars (keloids)

4. Constipation with no desire for bowel movements and large stools

Constipation following operations

Digestive problems with wind and bloating

Haemorrhoids with anal fissures

5. Frigidity. Vaginal discharge. Hot flushes before the menopause

6. Nosebleeds

Site of action
• The skin

• The intestinal system

• The female reproductive system

• Endocrine regulation

Related remedies
Calcarea carbonica

Sensitive type
The person is fat and suffers with anaemia, constipation, and problems with the digestion. He or she is very sensitive to the cold. The skin is unhealthy and thickened. There is sadness and anxiety, and the person is sensitive to all impressions.

Gratiola
Source of the remedy
The whole plant Hedge Hyssop, when in bloom

Main actions
Explosive diarrhoea followed by exhaustion and anal irritation (especially in children)

Homeopathy encyclopedia

Modalities
Aggravated by hot weather and cold drinks

Site of action
The intestines

Related remedies

Gambogia, China, Aloe, Croton riglium, and Arsenicum album

Grindelia
Source of the remedy
The leaves and unopened flowers of the Rosin-Wood, known as the Gum Plant

Main actions
The sensation of suffocation on falling asleep and waking up. This remedy is used to treat asthma and fluid in the lung, but only as a complement to medical treatment.

Site of action
The heart and lungs

Related remedies

Lachesis and Aralia racemosa

Hamamelis virginiana
Hamamelis in brief
Remedy for disorders of the veins

Source of the remedy
The dry bark of the Witch Hazel shrub

Main actions
Varicose veins with inflammation and pain; haemorrhage of dark blood that does not clot easily

Secondary signs
Bruising after the slightest injury; nosebleeds; dilated veins, painful and sensitive to the touch; bleeding between periods

Modalities
Aggravated by heat

Suggested uses
1. Varicose veins and haemorrhoids

2. Bruising after trauma and subconjunctival haemorrhages (bruising on the whites of the eyes)

Site of action
The veins

Related remedies

Arnica, Aesculus, and Pulsatilla

Hecla lava
Source of the remedy
The finest ash of the lava from Mount Hecla in Iceland

Suggested uses
Remedy for all abnormal bony outgrowths (exostoses), especially in arthritis. Spurs of the heel bone

Site of action
The bones

Related remedies

Silica and Calcarea fluorica

Hedra helix
Source of the remedy
The Common Ivy

Main actions
Fatigue, feeling vaguely unwell, sensitivity to cold with constant state of anxiety and worry. Emotionally labile. Irregular periods

Site of action
The general health

Related remedies

Pulsatilla

Helianthus
Source of the remedy
The ripe seeds of the Sunflower

Main actions
Enlargement of the spleen and recurrent fever. This remedy is very little used. It is helpful for elderly people suffering with chronic malaria.

Site of action
• The spleen

• The immune system

Helleborus niger
Source of the remedy
The root of the Christmas Rose

Suggested uses
1. Deep depression with fixed ideas

2. Coma after a serious disease or trauma

3. This remedy can only be used as a complement, and is not a replacement for expert medical attention

Site of action

• The mental state

• The general health

Related remedies

Bufo rana

Helonias
Source of the remedy
The root of the False Unicorn plant, at the end of the flowering period

Main actions
Depression in women obsessed with gynaecological problems: prolapse of the uterus, vaginal discharges, and painful, sensitive, and hardened breasts before periods

Site of action
• The mental state

• The female reproductive system

Related remedies

Thuja and Sepia

Hepar sulph
Hepar sulph in brief
Excellent remedy for stimulating the immune system

Source of the remedy
Developed by Hahnemann, this remedy is prepared by burning a mixture of equal parts of Flowers of Sulphur and powdered Oyster Shell. The end result is an impure calcium sulphate.

Homeopathy encyclopedia

Main actions
Inflammation and infections of the skin, soft tissues, and glands. Increased sensitivity of the nervous system

Secondary signs
Boils; laryngitis with a hoarse, painful cough accompanied by sweating; enlarged pus-filled tonsils; swollen glands in the neck

Modalities
• Aggravated by dry cold, by the slightest touch

• Improved by heat

Use in 6C potency for conditions where pus is present

Site of action
• The immune system

• The skin and soft tissues

Sensitive type

This remedy is useful in all individuals. However, it is particularly appropriate for highly sensitive types, very sensitive to the cold and to pain, who are highly susceptible to infections.

Histamine
Source of the remedy
Histamine Hydrochloricum

Suggested uses
All allergies, particularly eczema, asthma, and allergic rhinitis

Site of action
The immune system

Hura brasilensis
Source of the remedy
The sap of the Hura Brasilensis tree

Main actions
Inflammation and irritation in the rectum and anus. Eruptions of blisters on skin covering prominent bones such as the cheekbones

Site of action
• The rectum

• The skin

Related remedies

Sulphur, Nitric acid, Paeonia, and Mercurius corrosivus

Hydrastis
Source of the remedy
The roots of the Golden Seal herb

Main actions
Thick, yellow secretions from the soft tissues of the nose, pharynx, sinuses, larynx, respiratory systems and urinary systems. Liver and digestive complaints. Weight loss. General ill health

Modalities
Aggravated by cold, by eating bread and vegetables, and by laxatives

Site of action
The soft tissues, especially those of the respiratory system

Related remedies

Kali bichromicum, Berberis vulgaris, Arsenicum album, and Thuja

Hydrocyanic acid

Source of the remedy
Dilute Hydrocyanic Acid (Prussic acid), a very toxic substance

Main actions
Spasms in the oesophagus (gullet) making it impossible to swallow anything. Serious problems with the heart and lungs. Convulsions. This remedy is only really used for oesophageal spasms.

Site of action
• The heart and lungs

• The digestive system

Related remedies

Ignatia and Cuprum metallicum

Hyoscyamus niger

Hyoscyamus in brief
Remedy for children's nightmares

Source of the remedy
The black Henbane, whole and in bloom

Main actions
Mania with muscular spasms

Secondary signs
Acute mania alternating with phases of stupor. Exhibitionism; sexual excitement; dryness in the mucous membranes; insomnia

Modalities
• Aggravated by stretching out, by emotions, and fears

• Improved by sitting down and leaning forward

Suggested uses
1. Delirium, insomnia, nightmares (particularly in children)

2. Coughing spasms at night

Site of action
The central nervous system

Related remedies

Stramonium and Belladonna

Hypericum perforatum

Hypericum perforatum in brief
Major remedy for nerve pains, especially as a consequence of shingles

Source of the remedy
St. John's Wort, whole and in bloom

Main actions
Painful hypersensitivity of the nerve endings

Secondary signs
Sharp pains, which shoot along the course of the traumatized nerve

Modalities
Aggravated by touch and by jolting

Suggested uses
1. Any trauma affecting a nerve ending
2. Facial neuralgia, facial paralysis
3. Any recent trauma affecting the brain or spinal cord
4. Pain resulting from shingles
5. Painful scars

Homeopathy encyclopedia

Site of action
- The central nervous system
- The nerves

Related remedies

Kalmia

Ignatia

Ignatia in brief
- Major remedy (polychrest)
- For increased sensitivity to stimuli
- Anxiety
- Tendency to spasms and cramps
- Nervous conditions

Source of the remedy
The seeds of the St. Ignatius Bean

Main actions
Heightened senses (especially hearing); emotional sensitivity and instability; tendency to spasms; poor coordination

Secondary signs
Contradictory and paradoxical symptoms; sensation of a lump in the throat; anxiety leading to hurried behaviour; involuntary sighing; compulsive yawning; general feeling of weakness, pangs of hunger around 11 a.m.; sudden, fleeting pains; migraines as if a nail were being hammered into the head

Modalities
- Aggravated by emotions, grief, setbacks, in the morning around 11 a.m., by strong smells (tobacco, coffee, and perfume), consolation and overwork
- Improved by changing position, distraction, heat, and forceful pressure

Suggested uses
1. Remedy for nervous over-reactions in 'tortured souls', with countless symptoms that are constantly changing

2. Tendency to spasms

Site of action
- The central nervous system
- The mental state

Related remedies

Gelsemium, Staphysagria, and Pulsatilla

Sensitive type

The Ignatia personality is one who is anxious, impulsive, and emotionally unstable. He, or she, reacts in a disproportionate way to stress. A minor setback can provoke a nervous breakdown, yet the death of a loved one might only bring about a minor reaction.

They are often found in steady jobs, as civil servants, for example, because such work provides a haven of security.

There are no specific physical characteristics associated with the Ignatia type. These paradoxical mood changes can be seen in people of different body builds. It is also very common to find people of another constitutional type who, at certain times of their life, show similar behaviour patterns, but this does not mean that this remedy should be continually prescribed. Many people become distraught during difficult periods of change, and demonstrate the type of symptoms described above.

Influenzinum

Source of the remedy
The influenza virus

Suggested uses
Prevention of influenza and flu symptoms

Site of action
The immune system

Related remedies

Oscillococcinum

Iodium

Iodium in brief
Remedy for depression with anxiety

Source of the remedy
Iodine

Main actions
Weight loss despite a ferocious appetite, palpitations, trembling, anxiety, depression, hypersensitivity, and irritability

Modalities
• Aggravation from the heat and resting

• Better for eating, fresh air, and movement

Suggested uses
1. Depression following emotional upsets

2. Emotional, hypersensitive people with great anxiety

3. Spasmodic disorders: cough, colitis

Site of action
The central nervous system

Related remedies

Phosphorus and Ignatia

Sensitive type

The person is very thin despite a voracious appetite. He or she tires rapidly and cannot tolerate heat. He or she is anxious and depressed, and needs to be active in order to relieve anxiety.

Ipecacuanha (Ipecac)

Ipecac in brief
• Remedy for digestive and intestinal disorders with nausea and vomiting

• Spasmodic cough and acute bronchitis

Source of the remedy
The root of the shrub which bears the same name

Main actions
Intense nausea, vomiting, and diarrhoea; nasal discharge with continuous sneezing; suffocating cough. Difficulty in coughing up phlegm. Attacks of asthma. Haemorrhage of bright red blood from the digestive and respiratory systems

Ipecacuanha (Ipecac)

Secondary signs
Complaints recur, often at night. Clean tongue and intense salivation

Modalities
• Aggravated by movement and by variations in temperature

• Improved by resting and by pressure

Suggested uses
1. Indigestion with a moist, clean tongue and copious saliva

2. Absence of thirst. Aversion to all food. Despite the vomiting of abundant amounts of slimy vomit, severe nausea persists. Occasional vomiting of red blood

2. Colic with cramps around the navel. Nausea in pregnancy with excessive salivation

3. Inflammatory bowel disease with haemorrhages from the rectum or large bowel

4. Spasmodic cough with suffocation and nausea accompanied by vomiting (an indication in whooping cough). Acute bronchitis with abundant mucus in the chest. Asthma that recurs regularly every year, with nausea and vomiting

Site of action
• The digestive system

• The respiratory system

• The central nervous system

Related remedies

Antimonium tartaricum, Cuprum, Euphrasia, and Cocculus

Iris tenax
Source of the remedy
The rhizome of the Iris Minor plant

Suggested uses
1. Pain in the area of the appendix, appendicitis

2. Post-operative pains (appendectomy)

3. A minor remedy, but very effective in these cases

Site of action
The appendix

Related remedies

Bryonia and Opium

Iris versicolor
Source of the remedy
The fresh rhizome of the Blue Flag iris

Main actions
Burning throughout the digestive tract; reflux of the stomach contents into the mouth; burning diarrhoea; migraines with visual disturbances, nausea, and vomiting, recurring on a weekly basis

Site of action
The circulation and the digestive tract

Related remedies

Sulphur, Cyclamen, Gelsemium, and Robina

Jaborandi

Source of the remedy
The Pilocarpus plant used whole

Main actions
Excessive salivation, sweating, eye-strain

Related remedies

Ruta (for tired eyes)

Kali arsenicosum

Kali arsenicosum in brief
Minor remedy for eczema

Source of the remedy
Potassium Arsenate

Main actions
Dry skin rashes and fissures in the folds of the elbow and knees

Suggested uses
Eczema in an emaciated person who is sensitive to the cold and hates the open air. The eczema is similar in appearance to that found in Arsenicum album states.

Site of action
The skin

Related remedies

Arsenicum album and Arsenicum iodatum

Kali bichromicum (Kali bic)

Kali bichromicum in brief
• Major remedy for the digestive and respiratory systems

• The skin

• The joints

Source of the remedy
Potassium Bichromate

Main actions
Inflammation in the digestive and respiratory systems, with abundant, sticky, viscous, greenish-yellow mucus. Ear, nose, and throat infections with pus

Deep, punched out ulcers in the nose, mouth, and stomach

Various skin rashes with deep ulcers. Joint pains

Secondary signs
Alternation of recurrent complaints, e.g. rheumatism alternating with intestinal disorders. Well-localized pains that continually move from place to place

Modalities
• Aggravated by the cold, by drinking beer (although this is enjoyed), at around 3 a.m.

• Improved by heat

Suggested uses
1. Mouth ulcers. Stomach ulcers. Headaches with digestive problems. Migraines located at the root of the nose

2. Acute nasal discharges. Sinusitis in the forehead or cheek bones. Ulcerating tonsillitis

3. Lumbago. Sciatica. Pains in the heel. Pains in the tendons

Kali bichromicum

4. Certain types of eczema. Impetigo. Varicose ulcers

5. Infections of the uterus with thick greenish discharge

Site of action
• Ear, nose, and throat, and the mouth

• The skin

• The joints

Related remedies

Mercurius vivus, Hydrastis, Hepar sulph, and Thuja

Sensitive type

Plump subject who appears to be bursting with health

Kali bromatum

Kali bromatum in brief
Remedy for childhood psychological disorders and acne

Source of the remedy
Potassium Bromide

Main actions
Depression with memory loss. The person is restless, appears distracted and indifferent, and constantly gesticulates. Eruptions of acne on greasy skin, with hard, pustular spots on the face, back, and chest

Secondary signs
Insomnia in children, with night terrors; reduced sensitivity to pain

Modalities
• Aggravated at night, at the new moon, and by intellectual exertion

• Improved by physical activity

Suggested uses
1. Restless children who suffer night terrors and are behind at school. Memory disorders

2. Bed-wetting

3. Acne with pustules

Site of action
• The central nervous system

• The skin

Related remedies

Hyoscyamus, Kali phosphoricum, and Sulphur iodatum

Kali carbonicum

Source of the remedy
Potassium Carbonate

Main actions
Weakness, poor general health, sensitivity to the cold, and irritability

Multiple health problems: tired muscles, weak heart or kidneys leading to ankle swelling, catarrh, weak lungs, asthma, problems with digestion, haemorrhoids, urinary problems, period problems, anaemia and arthritis

Secondary signs
Abundant sweating, even in cold weather

Modalities
- Aggravated around 3 a.m., by damp cold, by the slightest exertion

- Improved by heat

Suggested uses
Major remedy for ageing and progressive organ failure

Site of action
The whole body

Related remedies

Natrum carbonicum, Arsenicum album, Sepia, Calcarea carbonica, and Psorinum

Sensitive type

This remedy is particularly indicated in depressed, discouraged, weary subjects who are hypersensitive to noise and being touched, even very lightly, and very upset by the slightest setback. The complexion is pale, the face is bloated, sometimes with a small characteristic sign: a swelling in the upper inner corner of the eyelid.

Kali iodatum
Source of the remedy
Potassium Iodide

Main actions
Acute and chronic nasal catarrh with irritating discharge, burning watery eyes, sinusitis in the forehead. Joint and bone pains (knees, heels and toes). Facial neuralgia

Modalities
- Aggravated by heat, at night

- Improved by fresh air, by movement

Site of action
- The linings of the nose, eyes, and sinuses

- The immune system (lymph glands)

- The joints

- The nerves

Related remedies

Iodum, Kali bichromicum, Sulphur and Euphrasia

Kali muriaticum
Source of the remedy
Potassium Chloride

Main actions
Tonsillitis: the tonsils are greyish white and ulcerated. Serious ear infections

Site of action
The immune system

Related remedies

Baryta carbonica

Kali nitricum
Kali nitricum in brief
Minor remedy for heart failure and asthma

Source of the remedy
Potassium Nitrate

Kali nitricum

Main actions
Oppressive pain in the chest, with great discomfort when breathing. Weak heart and slow pulse

Secondary signs
Sensation of coldness in the heart; weakness and abnormal sensitivity to the cold; slow, weak pulse; asthma in cold, damp weather

Modalities
Aggravated by damp cold

Suggested uses
1. Heart failure with a tendency to blackouts

2. Asthma

Site of action
The heart and lungs

Related remedies

Bryonia alba

Kali phosphoricum
Kali phosphoricum in brief
Remedy for physical and psychological weakness

Source of the remedy
Potassium Phosphate

Main actions
Great depression with nervous exhaustion. Muscular weakness. Anaemia

Secondary signs
Loss of memory, irritability, and emotional states. Headaches in school children and students. Insomnia after the slightest excitement. Vertigo and dizzy spells. Heightened sexual desire but reduced potency

Modalities
• Aggravated by intellectual work, sexual relationships, cold, and movement

• Improved by eating and being in company

Suggested uses
1. Physical and psychological weakness after overwork or excessive sexual activity. Impotence

2. Convalescence. Headaches and memory problems in students

3. Night terrors

Site of action
The central nervous system

The general health

Related remedies

Conium, Onosmodium and Ignatia.

Kali suphuricum
Source of the remedy
Potassium Sulphate

Suggested uses
Thick, yellow secretions, which do not irritate, especially in the final stages of an infectious disease

Site of action
The immune system

Related remedies

Pulsatilla

Kalmia latifolia

Kalmia Latifolia in brief
Remedy for violent neuralgia

Source of the remedy
The leaf of the Mountain Laurel tree

Main actions
Rheumatic pains that shift from one site to another. Very painful neuralgia that shoots along the length of the nerve, often on the face and around the eye

Secondary signs
Heart pain with a weak, slow pulse

Modalities
Aggravated by movement, during the early part of the night

Suggested uses
1. Violent neuralgia in the form of shooting pains: sciatica, facial neuralgia and pelvic pain

2. Neuralgia following shingles

Site of action
The nerves

Related remedies

Hypericum

Kreosotum

Source of the remedy
Creosote, a product distilled from wood tar

Main actions
Early dental caries with extensive decay. Irritating, foul-smelling, bloody discharges and ulceration in the genitals, urinary and digestive tracts.

Site of action
• The teeth

• The linings of the body cavities (mucosa)

Related remedies

Carbo animalis, Arsenicum album, and Causticum

Lac caninum

Lac caninum in brief
Minor remedy for swollen breasts during the menstrual cycle

Source of the remedy
The milk of a Female Dog. Remedy for the breast, when the symptoms alternate from one side to the other.

Main actions
Swelling and hardening of the breasts. Tendency for the symptoms to alternate from one side to the other

Suggested uses
1. Swelling and pains in the breasts at certain times in the menstrual cycle

2. All illnesses that start on one side of the body then move to the other side

Site of action
The breasts

Lachesis

Lachesis in brief
• Major remedy (polychrest)

Homeopathy encyclopedia

- For venous disorders

- Menopause

- Jealousy and heightened senses

Source of the remedy
Venom from a South American snake

Main actions
Disturbances of the heart rate and respiration. Problems with the blood vessels, which are either too dilated or constricted. The blood clots less well, leading to haemorrhages and bruises.

Secondary signs
Left-sided symptoms. Great sensitivity to heat, noise, and, above all, to being touched. Excitation alternating with depression. Loquacity. Jealousy. Inability to sleep before midnight. Distressing dreams of death. Dry tongue. Purple discoloration of the tonsils, which are acutely painful. Swallowing very painful, especially for liquids. Purplish external piles, that improve after bleeding

Craving for alcohol and oysters. Sinusitis or nasal catarrh, that starts with headaches and is improved by discharges. Hot flushes. Congestive headaches

Migraines, especially left-hand sided. High blood pressure. Problems with varicose veins and the veins. Irregular periods, which are slightly heavy with a flow of black blood

Modalities
All the problems are improved when a period starts

Suggested uses
1. Major remedy for the menopause and problems associated with it

2. All disorders of the veins

3. Alcoholism, alcoholic delirium

4. Psychological disorders: jealousy, persecution complex

Site of action
- The central nervous system

- The mental state

- The female reproductive system

- The veins

Related remedies

Vipera, Ignatia, Sepia, and Nux vomica

Sensitive type

The Lachesis person is emotionally unstable, and over-reacts. He, or she, is overly sensitive and lacks trust, believing that everyone is out to get them. They are very loquacious and hop from one subject to another. Their words come out in torrents.

There is, however, another hidden side. These are very active people, who worry a great deal and rush around. When faced with the realization that a task is beyond them, the normal reserve vanishes. They explode into anger, swearing at anyone who refuses to comply with their demands for help.

They are usually middle-aged women, on the plump side. The face is usually full, and can be blotchy if they are heavy drinkers. However, people of both sexes and all ages and body types may respond to Lachesis.

Lachnantes tinctoria

Lachnantes tinctoria in brief
Minor remedy for pain and stiffness in the neck

Source of the remedy
The whole plant of the same name

Main actions
Pains in the head and the back of the neck; sore throat

Suggested uses
Pain and stiffness in the neck, especially on the right-hand side

Site of action
The neck and neck bones

Related remedies

Cimicifuga

Lactic acid

Source of the remedy
Lactic acid

Suggested uses
Nausea in pregnancy with excessive salivation

Site of action
The autonomic nervous system (the part of the nervous system that regulates bodily functions on a sub-conscious level)

Lapis albus

Lapis albus in brief
• Good remedy for uterine fibroids

• All benign tumours of the glands

Source of the remedy
Calcium Silico-Fluorica

Main actions
Swollen, rubbery glands

Site of action
1. All benign swellings of the glandular tissues that are soft and rubbery

Thyroid and breast tumours, those in the female reproductive system, especially fibroids

2. Thyroid goitres

Site of action
• The female reproductive system

• The endocrine glands

Related remedies

Fraxinus americana

Latrodectus mactans

Source of the remedy
The Black Widow spider (usually the female) used whole

Suggested uses
Pains in the heart, angina pectoris, and myocardial infarction

This remedy is only used today as a complement to conventional medical treatment.

Site of action
The cardiovascular system

Related remedies

Aconite, Lachesis, Naja, and Carbo vegetabilis

Laurocerasus
Source of the remedy
The leaves of the Cherry Laurel tree

Suggested uses
Spasms in the throat, larynx, and oesophagus. Heart failure

This remedy must be used as a complement to conventional medical treatment

Site of action
The autonomic nervous system (the part of the nervous system that regulates bodily functions on a subconscious level)

Ledum palustre
Ledum palustre in brief
• For the treatment of traumas and insect bites

• Gout

Source of the remedy
The leafy branches of the Marsh tea plant

Main actions
Acute, sub-acute, or chronic inflammations of the small joints. Purplish bruises, especially on the limbs. Dry skin rashes and itching

Secondary signs
Rheumatism that starts at the feet and works its way upwards

Modalities
• Aggravated by movement, by heat, and at night

• Improved by resting and by cold

Suggested uses
1. Bruises in general (after Arnica) and, particularly, trauma to the eye

2. Penetrating wounds from a sharp object such as a nail

3. Insect bites (in alternation with Apis mellifica)

4. Gout in the big toe. Painful sensitive soles of the feet

5. Acne rosacea in alcoholics

6. Old, painful ulcers

Site of action
The veins

Related remedies

Arnica, Apis mellifica, Aesculus, and Hamamelis

Leptandra virginica
Source of the remedy
The fresh root of the plant known as Black Root

Main actions
Pitch-black diarrhoea caused by disease of the liver, aggravated by cold drinks, improved by lying on the stomach

Warning
Black diarrhoea is a sign of internal bleeding from the digestive tract. A full medical examination and appropriate investigations are essential to find the source. However, homeopathic treatment can be used while waiting for the results of the tests.

Site of action
The liver and the digestive system

Related remedies

Arsenicum album

Lilium tigrinum
Lilium tigrinum in brief
Minor remedy for fibroids and the menopause

Source of the remedy
The Tiger Lily, whole and in bloom

Main actions
Deep depression with severe irritability. Heaviness in the pelvis, frequent desire for urination or bowel movements. Light periods, with blood clots that only appear in times of activity. Ovarian pains on the left-hand side

Secondary signs
Religious mania and high sex drive, that leads to feelings of guilt

Modalities
• Aggravation from heat, resting, lying on the right-hand side, and from consolation

• Improved by the open air, by lying on the left-hand side, by keeping busy

Suggested uses
1. Congestion of the uterus and the ovaries. Uterine fibroids

2. Problems related to the menopause

3. Psychological problems and a high sex drive

Site of action
• The female reproductive system

• The central nervous system

Related remedies

Lapis albus, Fraxinus americana, and Thuja

Lithium carbonicum
Source of the remedy
Lithium Carbonate

Main actions
Raised uric acid levels, gout, pains in the small joints in the hands

Site of action
The skeletal system

Related remedies

Lycopodium and Actea spicata

Lobelia inflata
Source of the remedy
The whole, fresh Puke-Weed plant when in bloom

Main action
Intense nausea with a tendency to fainting, breathing difficulties, asthma with heart disease

Homeopathy encyclopedia

Site of action
The autonomic nervous system (the part of the nervous system that regulates bodily functions on a subconscious level).

Related remedies

Tabacum, Ipecac, and Cocculus

Lueticum (Syphilinum)
Lueticum in brief
Major remedy for all destructive lesions

Source of the remedy
Remedy made from the fluid from a Syphilitic lesion

Main actions
Syphilis causes inflammation, ulceration, and then tissue destruction and scarring. The remedy is used where the disease process follows this pattern.

Suggested uses
Many uses but only in the hands of a professional homeopath

Site of action
General health and the immune system

Lycopodium
Lycopodium in brief
• Major remedy (polychrest)

• For liver problems

• Digestive disorders

• Enlargement of the prostate

• An authoritarian and anxious person

Source of the remedy
The dry spores of the plant known as Club Moss

Main actions
Diseases of the liver, with shrinkage of the organ. Slow digestion with abdominal bloating after meals. Kidney and bladder stones, and high levels of uric acid. Impotence. Dry, wrinkled skin. Physical and psychological weakness

Depression, with preservation of intellectual powers

Secondary signs
Right-sided complaints, may shift to the left side. Sullen, sad, and irritable person. Voracious hunger. Craving for sweet things and oysters. Intolerance of onions. Very sensitive scalp

Modalities
• Aggravated by waking up, between 4 and 8 p.m., by heat, being contradicted, fatty substances, cold, heat

• Improved by movement, fresh air, hot food and drink

Suggested uses
1. Slow digestion with flatulence in a person with lower abdominal swelling. Stomach or duodenal ulcer with burning in the oesophagus. Gallstones. Vomiting and lack of appetite in children due to sugar intolerance

2. Kidney stones. Enlargement of the prostate with difficulties in passing urine. Impotence, despite normal sexual desire

3. Dry, wrinkled skin, with foul-smelling sweat. Hair prematurely grey. Chronic urticaria (hives)

4. Vaginal dryness in the menopause

5. Migraines, often in the right forehead and associated with digestive disorders, sometimes with problems with the eyesight

Site of action
• The liver

• The digestive tract

• The skin

• The nervous system

• The prostate

Related remedies

Berberis vulgaris, Chelidonium, Nux vomica, and Aurum metallicum

Sensitive type

The constitutional Lycopodium is anxious but ambitious, with great determination. He, or she, gives the impression of having great self-control.

They appear reserved and impassive: their pride prevents them from showing their emotional sensitivity. They act condescendingly or scornfully to anyone who dares to contradict them. They explode into violent rages of indignation, and turn livid with anger.

They are usually thin with poorly developed musculature. The chest is narrow

and the abdomen distended, as a result of their digestive problems.

These strange characters have one outstanding feature: their sharp, penetrating, almost accusatory, gaze, which is noticeable at birth and always makes the children appear older than their years.

Lycopus virginicus
Source of the remedy
The whole Bugleweed when in bloom

Suggested uses
Palpitations and increased heart rate in a person with an over-active thyroid gland

Site of action
The autonomic nervous system (the part of the nervous system that regulates bodily functions on a sub-conscious level)

Related remedies

Iodium, Lachesis, Spigelia, and Ignatia

Magnesia carbonica
Source of the remedy
Magnesium Carbonate

Main actions
Neuralgic pains running the length of the nerve; excess stomach acid; diarrhoea; painful periods with black blood; flow only occurs at night

Secondary signs
Neuralgia of the facial and dental

nerves; sensory disturbances; cramps in the limbs

Modalities
• Aggravated at night, by milk, by cold

• Improved by walking, in the open air, by local heat

• Health problems recur with regularity (often every three weeks)

Suggested uses
1. Nervousness and tendency to cramps

2. Diarrhoea in a baby, especially with milk intolerance

3. Period problems, with cramps and discharge of black blood

Site of action
• The nervous system

• The digestive system

• The female reproductive system

Related remedies

Chamomilla and Magnesia phosphorica

Magnesia muriatica
Source of the remedy
Magnesium Chloride

Main actions
Pains in the area of the liver; constipation with very dry, hard stools; painful periods with headaches in the preceding days

Secondary signs
Cramping pains improved by strong

pressure; disturbances of the sensory system

Modalities
• Aggravated by immobility, the seaside, milk, and salt

• Improved by movement, strong pressure, and the open air

Suggested uses
1. Constipation in a subject with pains in area of the liver and gall bladder

2. Painful periods with dark blood and clots

Site of action
• The digestive system and liver

• The female reproductive system

Related remedies

Silica, Lycopodium, and Thuja

Magnesia phosphorica
Magnesia phosphorica in brief
Major remedy for all muscle spasms

Source of the remedy
Magnesium Phosphate

Main actions
Painful cramping spasms in muscles, both in the internal organs and the skeletal system, starting and ending abruptly, and often moving to different parts of the body

Modalities
• Aggravated by cold

• Improved by heat, by doubling over

Suggested uses
All cramping pains: painful diarrhoea, period problems, facial neuralgia, cramps, kidney and gall bladder colic

Site of action
• The muscles

• The nerves

Colocynthis, Cuprum metallicum, and Cimicifuga

Manganum aceticum

Manganum in brief
Major remedy for fatigue

Source of the remedy
Manganese Acetate

Main actions
Fatigue and depression. Irritation in the upper airways with an almost permanent cold, constant hoarseness, and a cough in cold, damp weather. Laryngitis with pains that spread to the ear

Modalities
• Aggravated by humidity and cold, before a storm

• Improved by lying down

Suggested uses
Profound fatigue (use in 30C potency)

Site of action
The whole metabolism

Related remedies

Kali phosphoricum

Medorrhinum

Medorrhinum in brief
Major remedy (polychrest) for sycosis (as defined under Thuja), the tendency to rheumatism, repetitive pelvic infections, and restless behaviour

Source of the remedy
The discharges taken from the urethra of a person infected with Gonorrhoea, prior to any antibiotic treatment

Main actions
Chronic pelvic infections: infections of the urethra, prostate, ovaries, tubes, and chronic vaginal discharges. Subacute and chronic rheumatism. Impatient, restless behaviour

Secondary signs
Sciatica, especially on the left side. Pain and burning sensations on the hands and feet

Modalities
• Aggravated during the day, in cold, dry weather, by storms

• Improved by the seaside, by humidity, by friction

Suggested uses
1. All types of rheumatism

2. All after-effects of pelvic infections treated with antibiotics

3. Adverse reactions to vaccination and certain types of medication

4. Nasal catarrh, recurrent infections in the pharynx, ears, throat, and sinuses

Medorrhinum

5. Nappy rash

6. Warts

7. Sleep disorders in a restless child

8. Depression

Site of action
• The immune system

• General health

• The central nervous system

Related remedies

Thuja, Mercurius solubilis, Pulsatilla, Kali bichromicum, and Argentum nitricum

Sensitive type

Medorrhinum is a major remedy for sycosis (see Thuja) in all subjects. However, there is a type who is particularly sensitive to this remedy. This is a person, a child or an adult, who does everything in a hurry and behaves in an unstable, agitated, and anxious fashion.

Melilotsus officinalis
Source of the remedy
The whole fresh Sweet Clover plant, when in flower

Suggested uses
Congestive headaches relieved by a nosebleed or another haemorrhage. Sunstroke, with throbbing headaches

Modalities
• Aggravated in the menopause and by storms

• Improved by a haemorrhage

Site of action
The blood and the vascular system

Related remedies

Lachesis, Sulphur, and Aurum

Menyanthes
Source of the remedy
The Buckbean plant used whole and in bloom

Main actions
Fever or headaches with a feeling of intense cold

Site of action
The immune system

Related remedies

Camphora

Mephitis
Source of the remedy
The foul-smelling secretion from the Skunk's anal glands

Main actions
Troublesome cough (similar to whooping cough) with spasms in the larynx and a sensation of suffocation. Spasm when swallowing

Modalities
• Aggravated in bed at night

• Improved by cold baths

Site of action
The larynx and the trachea

Related remedies

Drosera, Corallium rubrum, Sambucus nigra, and Lachesis

Mercurius corrosivus

Mercurius corrosivus in brief
Major remedy for ulceration in the mucous membranes

Source of the remedy
Mercury Chloride (corrosive sublimate)

Main actions
Rapidly spreading ulceration on all the mucous membranes. Violent spasms in the internal organs, especially the bladder and rectum

Secondary signs
Ulceration in the throat, with intense burning sensation and great pain when swallowing. Mouth ulcers. Diarrhoea with burning, blood-streaked, foul-smelling stools. Constant, painful desire to open the bowels. Urinary infections with burning in the urethra. Very irritating vaginal discharge. Ulceration on the eyelids

Suggested uses
1. Serious gastro-enteritis

2. Ulcerative tonsillitis

3. Acute cystitis

4. Copious vaginal discharge

5. Acute conjunctivitis. Styes

Site of action
• All the membranes

• The immune system

Related remedies

Cantharis and Mercurius vivus

Mercurius cyanatus

Source of the remedy
Mercury Cyanide

Suggested uses
Diphtheria and severe cases of tonsillitis, with extreme fatigue

This remedy can only be used as a complement to classical treatments

Site of action
• The throat

• The immune system

Mercurius dulcis

Source of the remedy
Mercury Chloride

Suggested uses
• Middle ear infections with a clear discharge, following upper respiratory tract infections

• Diarrhoea in children

Site of action
• The ears

• The immune system

Related remedies

Ferrum phosphoricum

Mercurius iodatus flavus

Source of the remedy
An iodide of Mercury

Homeopathy encyclopedia

Suggested uses
Tonsillitis starting on the right side, that spreads towards the left

Site of action
• The throat

• The immune system

Related remedies

Lycopodium, Mercurius vivus, and Pulsatilla

Mercurius iodatus ruber
Source of the remedy
An iodide of Mercury

Suggested uses
Tonsillitis starting on the left side that spreads towards the right

Site of action
• The throat

• The immune system

Related remedies

Lachesis, Mercurius vivus, and Pulsatilla

Mercurius vivus
Mercurius vivus in brief
• Major remedy (polychrest)

• For infectious diseases in children

• Suppurative conditions (forming pus)

• Digestive disorders

• Urinary infections

• Severe health problems

Source of the remedy
Mercury (Quicksilver)

Main actions
Inflammation and ulceration in the digestive, genital, and urinary systems. Vomiting, copious amounts of diarrhoea, often bloody, and blood in the urine with reduced urine output. Foul breath. Swollen neck glands. Swollen tongue that bears the imprint of the teeth, with a yellow coating. Excessive salivation. Severe health problems. Weakness with pallor and anaemia. Episodes of fever with shivering and trembling. Profuse sweating, especially at night. Tendency to pus-forming conditions

Secondary signs
Impulsive, anxious, and depressed people; increase in all secretions and excretions, which are offensive; superficial ulceration which spreads rapidly

Modalities
• Aggravated at night, by extremes of temperature, the damp, weather changes, and by sweating

• Improved by rest, dry heat, and moderate temperatures

Suggested uses
1. Inflammatory and infectious conditions of the mouth, tonsils, upper respiratory tract, and glands. Mumps. Gastro-enteritis. Boils in the ear canal

2. Acute cystitis

3. Vaginal infections and discharges

Site of action
• The digestive system

• The upper respiratory tract

• The bladder

• The immune system

Related remedies

Belladonna, Mercurius corrosivus, and Argentum nitricum

Sensitive type

The constitutional Mercury type is slow, both physically and mentally, and is not very active. He, or she, is restless and trembling, inhibited, and pale and sweaty.

However, Mercurius vivus can be used for the appropriate conditions in all sorts of people, even if they do not show the constitutional picture.

Mezerium
Source of the remedy
The bark from the tree known as the Daphne Mezerium)

Main actions
Neuralgia with sensory disturbances, extreme sensitivity to touch. Neuralgia following shingles. Facial neuralgia. Itchy blistering rashes with pustules

Maxillary sinusitis with an irritating, burning discharge

Modalities
Aggravated at night, by the heat of the bed, by damp cold, and by the disappearance of the rash

Site of action
• The nerves

• The immune system

• The skin

Related remedies

Kalmia, Chamomilla, and Staphysagria

Millefolium
Millefolium in brief
An excellent remedy for all haemorrhages

Source of the remedy
The whole Yarrow plant when in bloom

Main actions
Painless haemorrhages of red blood, without anxiety

Suggested uses
Spontaneous or traumatic haemorrhages, in any location: nose, larynx, lungs, mouth, stomach, intestines, kidneys, bladder, uterus

Site of action
The blood and the veins

Related remedies

Arnica and Ledum palustre

Mixed pollens and grasses
Source of the remedy
Pollens from various Flowers and Grasses

Homeopathy encyclopedia

Suggested uses
Allergies, especially hay fever

Site of action
The immune system

Related remedies

Histamine

Momordica balsamina
Source of the remedy
The fresh fruit of the Balsam apple

Suggested uses
Pain in the left upper abdomen caused by an accumulation of gas in the bowel

Site of action
The large bowel

Related remedies

Raphanus and Lycopodium

Morbillinum
Source of the remedy
The Measles virus

Suggested uses
This nosode is used for ailments following measles infection. It must never be used during an attack of measles.

Site of action
The immune system

Moschus
Moschus in brief
Major remedy for hysteria

Source of the remedy
Musk: a glandular secretion from the Musk Deer

Main actions
Increased sensitivity, spasms (lump in the throat, tendency to suffocation and fainting), and sexual excitement

Secondary signs
Tendency to faint; weeping alternating with hysterical laughter; constant need to breathe in deeply

Modalities
• Aggravated by the cold

• Improved by open air and massage

Suggested uses
1. All symptoms of hysteria

2. Heightened sexual excitement in women

3. Period problems of nervous origin, accompanied by fainting

Site of action
• The central nervous system

• The female reproductive system

Related remedies

Platina and Murex

Murex purpureus
Murex in brief
Remedy for increased sexuality in women

Source of the remedy
The Purple fish, a type of shellfish

Main actions
Congestion of the female reproductive organs, with increased sexual excitement

Secondary signs
Heaviness in the pelvis; thick vaginal discharge; short periods

Suggested uses
1. Pelvic congestion with increased sexual excitement

2. Problems with periods and the female hormones

Site of action
The female reproductive system

Related remedies

Moschus and Lilium tigrinum

Muriatic acid
Source of the remedy
Hydrochloric Acid

Main actions
Allergy to the sun, with severe inflammation of the skin. Dry mouth with ulcers. Inflammation of the anus, haemorrhoids that hurt with the slightest contact

Modalities
Aggravated by touch and sunshine

People who are very sensitive to the sun can take this remedy as a preventive before summer holidays.

Site of action
The skin and the membranes

Related remedies

Sulphur

Mygale
Source of the remedy
The Black Cuban spider used whole

Main actions
Muscular twitching, especially in the face, uncontrolled movements, and muscular spasms

Site of action
The central nervous system

Related remedies

Tarentula hispanica, Agaricus muscarius, Kali bromatum and Cuprum metallicum

Myristica
Source of the remedy
The sap from the bark of a tree found in Brazil

Main actions
Abscesses and whitlows; the remedy speeds up the formation, gathering, and elimination of pus

Site of action
The immune system

Related remedies

Hepar sulph, Pyrogen, and Calendula.

Naja
Source of the remedy
The venom of the Cobra

Main actions
Constricting chest pain, like that of angina pectoris, with disorders of the heart rate and respiratory problems. Throbbing headaches with pain in the temples. Pain in the left ovary. Depression with suicidal impulses combined with anxiety

Modalities
Aggravated at night, after sleeping and by lying on the left side

Site of action
• The heart

• The central nervous system

Related remedies

Aconite, Cactus grandiflorus, Lachesis, and Kalmia

Naphthaline
Naphthaline in brief
• Remedy for catarrh with frequent sneezing

• Cataracts

Source of the remedy
Naphthaline, the hydrocarbon extracted from Coal Tar

Main actions
Irritation of the lining of the respiratory tract. Clouding of the lens of the eye

Suggested uses
1. Frequent sneezing, watery eyes, and runny nose causing skin irritation. Asthma improved by exposure to air. Hay fever with watery eyes and runny nose, causing skin irritation

2. Cataracts

Site of action
• The nose and pharynx

• The eyes

Related remedies

Allium cepa, Euphrasia, and Calcarea fluorica

Natrum carbonicum
Natrum carbonicum in brief
• Remedy for depression

• Explosive diarrhoea

• Repeated sprains

Source of the remedy
Sodium Carbonate

Main actions
Mental and psychological weakness, with depression. Sensitivity to the cold. Extreme sensitivity to sensory stimuli. Nutritional disorders with muscular and joint weakness. Flatulence. Explosive, orange-yellow diarrhoea set off by milk and starchy food

Secondary signs
Headaches follow the least mental effort. Weak joints

Modalities
• Aggravated by heat and cold, the sun, stormy weather, the full moon, mental activity, noise, and music. Worse at 5 a.m. and 11 p.m.

• Improved by movement

Suggested uses
1. Depression as described above

2. Diarrhoea in a hot climate, caused by intolerance of heat or sunstroke

3. Repeated sprains with slight swelling of the ankle

Site of action
• The central nervous system

• The bowels

• The joints

Related remedies

Staphysagria, Calcarea fluorica, Lachesis, Iodum, and Kali phosphoricum

Sensitive type

The person is overweight, and suffers with profound depression

Natrum muriaticum
Natrum muriaticum in brief
• Major remedy (polychrest)

• For nutritional problems. Weight loss

• Physical and mental weakness. Convalescence

• Eczema. Warts. Acne

• Puberty in boys

• Depression

Source of the remedy
Sea Salt (Sodium Chloride)

Main actions
Nutritional problems, loss of weight in the upper part of the body, excess gastric acid, and anaemia. Dry mouth, throat, bowel, and vagina. Excessive discharges like egg white. Dry skin with areas of greasiness. Depression

Secondary signs
Mental and physical weakness, irritability. Abnormal craving for salt. Great thirst for small amounts of water. Hearty appetite, often without putting on any weight

Modalities
• Aggravated by consolation, heat, sun, around 10 a.m., by the seaside, intellectual work in the summer, and excessive salt intake

• Improved by open air, sweating

Suggested uses
1. Weight loss and weakness. Convalescence from acute or debilitating diseases. Dehydration

2. Some types of eczema on the scalp, along the hairline, and in the folds of the knees and elbows. Herpes following acute illnesses. Chronic urticaria. Warts on the knuckles and the palms of the hand. Some types of teenage acne

2. Depression leading to health problems. Disappointment in love. Problems with school work. Headaches in school children

3. Problems with digestion with constipation

4. Hay fever. Some types of asthma. Recurrent upper respiratory tract infections in children

Homeopathy encyclopedia

Site of action
- The general health

- Problems related to nutrition

- The skin

- The immune system

- The mental state

Related remedies

Sepia, Silica, Gelsemium, and Ignatia

Sensitive type

The Natrum muriaticum character is emotional, prone to anxiety, and morose rather than depressed. He, or she, is clumsy and irritable, and pushes other people away. There is great difficulty in communication, although they are very receptive to what they are told. They generally live in a state of mild depression from childhood, which makes them very sensitive.

They are thin and bony, despite a hearty appetite, and they have dry skin and brittle, lacklustre hair.

Natrum sulphuricum
Natrum sulphuricum in brief
- Remedy for gastro-enteritis, bronchitis, and other chest complaints, aggravated by the damp

- Joint problems, head and back injuries

Source of the remedy
Sodium Sulphate

Main actions
Digestive and respiratory problems; stiff joints; warts; depression

Secondary signs
Thick, yellowish, irritating discharges. Brown coated tongue with a bitter taste in the mouth. Itching when getting undressed. Bloated stomach with colic and diarrhoea in the morning, particularly after breakfast. Great thirst for very cold drinks. Aversion to meat and bread

Modalities
- Aggravated by the damp and humidity

- Improved by dry weather, after clearing the bowels, and by changing position

Suggested uses
1. Gastro-enteritis with watery diarrhoea expelled in spurts, with abundant wind. Constipation alternating with diarrhoea

2. Chest complaints aggravated by the damp, with abundant, thick, greenish-yellow phlegm and a characteristic pain in the base of the lung. Asthma with phlegm

3. Joint pains aggravated by the damp, mainly in the lower back, the knees, the right hip, and the ankles

4. The after-effects of head and back injuries

5. Skin problems including blisters

6. Depression

Site of action
- The respiratory system

- The digestive system

- The central nervous system

- The joints

Related remedies

Natrum carbonicum, Dulcamara, Rhus toxicodendron, Ruta, and Arnica

Sensitive type

These people are overweight, and prone to cellulite, particularly on the abdomen, buttocks, and thighs. They are indolent and slow. They are sad, depressed, and very sensitive to damp cold weather.

Niccolum metallicum

Source of the remedy
The metal Nickel

Main actions
Migraines and neuralgia in people suffering from nervous exhaustion. Spasms in the larynx and the trachea, with coughing

Modalities
- Aggravated by lying down and after waking up, until midday

- Improved by the open air and after eating when suffering with a headache

Site of action
The nervous system

Related remedies

Phosphorus, Zincum, and Manganum

Nitric acid

Source of the remedy
A solution of Nitric Acid

Main actions
Ulcers, fissures, and burning pain at the junction of skin and the mucous membranes

Secondary signs
Depression and irritability; pricking pains; weakness and extreme sensitivity to the cold; irritating discharges; warts

Modalities
- Aggravated by the cold and noise

- Improved by movement (in a car or train)

Suggested uses
1. Anal fissures

2. Eczema with fissures. Warts that bleed easily

3. Mouth ulcers

Site of action
- The junction of skin and mucous membranes

- The mouth

Related remedies

Antimonium crudum, Kali Bichromicum, and Argentum nitricum

Nux moschata

Nux moschata in brief
Remedy for depression and weakness, with a tendency to fainting

Homeopathy encyclopedia

Source of the remedy
Nutmeg

Main actions
Depression with profound drowsiness and lethargy, and a tendency to fainting. Great dryness in the skin and membranes

Secondary signs
Abrupt mood swings; significant abdominal swelling; great sensitivity to the cold

Modalities
• Aggravated by the damp cold, any exertion, and by strong emotions

• Improved by heat

Suggested uses
Weakness with a tendency to fainting, especially in people with digestive disorders, constipation and abdominal bloating

Site of action
• The central nervous system

• The digestive system

Related remedies

Nux vomica

Nux vomica
Nux vomica in brief
• Major remedy (polychrest)
• For states of excitation
• High blood pressure
• Digestive disorders
• Migraines

• Sedentary lifestyle

Source of the remedy
The seed of the Poison Nut tree

Main actions
Increased sensations, rapidly followed by convulsions. Increased excitation of the nervous system and the nerve supply of the bowel

Secondary signs
Irritable, quarrelsome and impulsive, particularly foul tempered first thing in the morning. Sleepiness after meals, improved by a short nap. Craving for alcohol, spicy food, and coffee. Aversion to bread and meat. Migraines from overindulgence at mealtimes. Liver problems. Constipation and haemorrhoids. Early morning wakening between 3 and 4 a.m. Bouts of sneezing in the morning. Runny nose during the day, which is blocked at night

Modalities
• Aggravated in the morning after getting up, after meals, by anger, intellectual effort, by coffee, wine, alcohol, and tobacco

• Improved by uninterrupted sleep, heat, damp weather, and short naps

Suggested uses
1. Increased sensitivity. Insomnia and memory problems after overworking. Migraines in sedentary people

2. High blood pressure in Nux vomica types

3. Cramps and convulsions

4. Problems with digestion after overindulgent eating. Constipation. Haemorrhoids. Alcoholism

5. Allergic rhinitis. Influenza with fever

Site of action
• The central nervous system

• The emotional state

• The digestive system

• The liver

Related remedies

Ignatia, Gelsemium, Sulphur, and Nux moschata

Sensitive type

These people are domineering, hyperactive, ambitious, aggressive, quarrelsome, pernickety, and excessive in everything to the point of greed. They are highly adaptable, providing that they can maintain their equilibrium. They are sedentary subjects who deliberately abuse coffee, wine, spirits, and tobacco on a regular basis.

A typical example is the company boss who is always snowed under with work, often a 'self-made man' in a responsible position but without any formal qualifications.

They are ruddy, and often a little overweight as a result of overeating and a sedentary lifestyle.

Oleander

Source of the remedy
The leaves of the Oleander plant

Main actions
Impetigo and eczema, often situated behind the ears, which weep fluid. Both urinary and faecal incontinence. Laziness with intellectual fatigue

Site of action
The immune system

Related remedies

Graphites, Mezereum, and Agaricus muscarius

Onosmodium
Onosmodium in brief
• Minor remedy for impotence and frigidity

• Pains in the eyes due to glaucoma

Source of the remedy
The root and fruit of the plant known as the False Cromwell

Main actions
Congestion and spasms in the female pelvic organs and swollen breasts. Pain moving the eyeballs and headaches after eyestrain or as a result of undetected long-sightedness. Problems with movement, particularly in the eyes and lower limbs. Problems with coordination. Impotence, with diminished libido (sexual desire), and frigidity

Modalities
• Aggravated by working too hard at school, by reading, and by darkness

• Improved by rest and sleep

Suggested uses
1. Painful eye movements. Remedy for

Homeopathy encyclopedia

certain types of glaucoma (only when prescribed by a professional homeopath)

2. Loss of sexual desire, impotence, and frigidity in a depressed person, with problems of coordination

Site of action
- The sexuality, both male and female
- The eye
- The central nervous system

Related remedies

Ruta, Conium, Sepia, and Agnus castus

Opium
Source of the remedy
The Opium Poppy

Main actions
Heightened senses, euphoria and vivid imagination. Sleepiness, feels no pain and wants for nothing. Strokes. Epilepsy. Severe constipation and paralysis of the bladder

Modalities
Aggravated by fear, heat and after sleeping

Site of action
The central nervous system

Related remedies

Gelsemium, Arnica, Nux vomica, Alumina, and Bryonia

Origanum
Origanum in brief
Remedy for heightened sexuality in young women

Source of the remedy
The whole marjoram plant, including the flowers

Main actions
Sexual excitement in young women, with erotic dreams and fantasies, itching on the breasts

Secondary signs
Frequent masturbation

Suggested uses
Craving for sexual relationships, with arousal and erotic dreams in girls or young women

Site of action
Sexuality in young women

Related remedies

Platina, Murex, and Lilium tigrinum

Oscillococcinum
Oscillococcinum in brief
Remedy for influenza, especially at the start

Suggested uses
This remedy is very effective in treating the early stages of influenza

Site of action
The immune system

Related remedies

Gelsemium, Eupatorium perfoliatum, and Bryonia

Oxalic acid
Source of the remedy
Oxalic Acid

Suggested uses

1. Kidney stones

2. Blue discoloration of the hands and legs

Modalities

Aggravated by food rich in oxalates: chocolate, coffee, sorrel, strawberries, spinach, and rhubarb

Site of action

• The urinary system

• The small blood vessels

Related remedies

Sulphur and Berberis

Paeonia

Source of the remedy
The root of the Peony plant

Main actions
Protruding inflammed haemorrhoids, with sharp, piercing pains. Anal fissures and fistulas

Site of action
Haemorrhoids

Related remedies

Aloe, Nitric acid, and Ratanhia

Palladium

Source of the remedy
The metal Palladium

Suggested uses
1. Acute pain in the right ovary

2. Proud character, with feelings of being unjustly treated

Modalities
• Aggravated by bad news

• Improved by firm pressure on the painful area and by everyday activity

Site of action
• The female reproductive system

• The emotional state

Related remedies

Platina, Staphysagria, Bryonia, and Lycopodium

Pareira brava

Pareira brava in brief
Remedy for kidney colic and urinary infections

Source of the remedy
The dry root of the Virgin Vine

Main actions
Kidney colic, kidney stones, and urinary infection

Secondary signs
Great effort required to urinate, in spite of a frequent urge to do so. Urinary infections in people prone to urine retention

Modalities
Improved by doubling over with the knees against the chest

Suggested uses
1. Kidney colic

2. Urinary infection in people with prostate problems, strictures or stones

Site of action
The urinary tract

The immune system

Berberis

Paris quadrifolia

Source of the remedy
The whole Paris Quadrifolia plant

Main actions
Headaches in the forehead and the eye sockets. Feeling as if the eyes are being pulled backwards. Painful, stiff neck. A stream of incoherent ramblings

Site of action
The nervous system

Lachnantes and Lachesis

Pertussin

Source of the remedy
The nosode of the whooping-cough bacterium

Suggested uses
For the ill effects of whooping cough, but only to be used by a homeopath

Site of action
• The immune system

• The respiratory system

Petroleum

Petroleum in brief
Remedy for cracks and fissures in the skin and for travel sickness

Source of the remedy
Crude Rock Oil

Main actions
Dry, thickened skin with irritation and dry cracked eczema. Cough and bronchitis. Visual disorders. Nausea and diarrhoea

Secondary signs
Skin problems alternating with digestive disorders. Sensitivity to cold and a sensation of coldness in parts of the body. Ravenous hunger, worse at night. Foul-smelling sweat in the armpits, groin, and feet. Vertigo and nausea when travelling, improved by closing the eyes

Modalities
• Aggravated by the cold, especially in winter, by cabbage and sauerkraut

• Improved by eating, the heat, and in the summer

Suggested uses
1. Chapped skin, fissures on the fingers, eczema

2. Diarrhoea following eating cabbage

3. Travel sickness

Site of action
• The inner ear

• The skin

• The digestive tract

Related remedies

Nitric acid and Cocculus

Phellandrium

Source of the remedy
The Water Dropwort plant

Suggested uses
Chronic bronchitis in smokers

Site of action
The immune system

Related remedies

Hepar sulph and Antimonium tartaricum

Phosphoric acid

Phosphoric acid in brief
• Remedy for serious depression

• Painless chronic diarrhoea

• Bone disorders in children and adolescents

Source of the remedy
Diluted Phosphoric Acid

Main actions
Depression with weakness. A tendency to withdraw from social situations, with a refusal to communicate, and indifference towards studying and exams. Night sweats. Sexual weakness after overindulgence. Painless diarrhoea with wind and undigested food. Decalcification of the bones

Secondary signs
Headaches on the top of the skull. Sleepiness in the day and insomnia at night, despite a great desire to go to sleep

Modalities
• Aggravated by emotional setbacks, overindulgence and noise. In the case of diarrhoea, by fruit

• Improved by sleep

Suggested uses
1. Depression with a retreat from the outside world, triggered by setbacks or profound grief

2. Painless, chronic diarrhoea that does not cause severe exhaustion

3. Growing pains in the bones

Site of action
• The central nervous system

• The intestines

Related remedies

Natrum carbonicum, Staphysagria, Kali phosphoricum, Calcarea phosphorica, and Silica.

Sensitive type

The typical Phosphoric acid type is a tall, thin adolescent who tires easily. He, or she, tends to get depressed and become indifferent to everything and everyone. He, or she, suffers with back problems, and chronic diarrhoea.

Phosphorus

Phosphorus in brief
• Major remedy (polychrest)

Phosphorus

• For haemorrhages and a bleeding tendency

• Inflammations of the liver (hepatitis), nerves, and kidneys (nephritis)

• Lung complaints

• Vertigo

• Increased sensitivity of the senses

Source of the remedy
Red Phosphorus

Main actions
Disorders of all the major organs, especially the liver, lungs, and kidneys. Loss of appetite, stomach pains, diarrhoea, and intestinal colic. Anxiety, restlessness, increased sensitivity, burning pains

Secondary signs
Tendency to haemorrhage. Congestion in the head and vertigo. Craving for salt and salty food. Craving for cold food and drink. Need to eat during the night

Modalities
Aggravated by any mental or physical exercise, strong emotions, solitude, overwork, during storms, at twilight, by cold, and by lying on the left-hand side

Suggested uses
1. Haemorrhage, whatever the cause

2. Liver problems, especially hepatitis and cirrhosis, and acute inflammations of the pancreas

3. Inflammation of the nerves caused by alcoholism

4. Lung infections, especially viral

5. Acute infections of the kidneys

6. Vertigo in elderly subjects

7. Weak heart

Site of action
• The liver

• The lungs

• The kidneys

• The nervous system

• The emotional state

Related remedies

Arsenicum album, Ferrum phosphoricum, and Lachesis

Sensitive type

These people, often artists, are dreamers who pay little attention to reality and live in the clouds. They are intuitive, imaginative, and highly emotional. They are impulsive. They are overly sensitive to noises, smells, light, and the atmosphere of particular places, and they adapt to life by retreating into an imaginary world. They always dress elegantly.

They are often tall and thin, with a long, slim chest. They often have triangular-shaped faces. Their skin is pale but flushes easily when they get excited.

Phytolacca decandra
Phytolacca in brief
• Major remedy for throat problems in singers, and for breast pain

• Suitable for some types of rheumatism

Source of the remedy
The whole plant, including the ripe fruits

Main actions
Inflammation of the throat; painful breasts; pain in the bones; rheumatism

Secondary signs
Bruised feeling; pain in the throat spreading up to the ears

Modalities
• Aggravated at night, by damp cold, and by movement

• Improved by lying down

Suggested uses
1. Sore throats in singers

2. Sore breasts before periods

3. Rheumatism

Site of action
• The throat

• The female reproductive system

• The joints

Related remedies

Ruta, Rhus toxicodendron, Belladonna, Mercurius vivus, Folliculinum, and Argentum nitricum

Picric acid

Picric acid in brief
Minor remedy for eczema in the auditory canal

Source of the remedy
Picric Acid

Main actions
Painful erection without any sexual desire (priapism) followed by nervous depression. Small boils

Suggested uses
1. Small boils found on eczema in the auditory canal

2. Priapism

Site of action
1. The auditory canal

2. The male reproductive system

Plantago

Source of the remedy
The Plantain plant, whole, when in bloom

Suggested uses
1. Bed-wetting in children (with very variable outcomes)

2. Painful teeth

Site of action
The nervous system

Related remedies

Natrum muriaticum and Opium

Platina

Platina in brief
• High sex drive

• Arrogance

• Cramps

• Constipation when travelling

Platina

Source of the remedy
The metal Platinum

Main actions
Physical and mental sexual excitement with increased sensitivity in the genital organs. Constrictive pains gradually come and go. Ovarian pains. Tendency to look down on other people. Constipation while travelling

Secondary signs
Haughtiness, arrogance

Modalities
• Aggravated by being touched, by pressure, fear, and celibacy

• Improved by walking

Suggested uses
1. Sexual excitement, especially in women

2. Cramps, spasms, and neuralgia, particularly during painful periods

3.Constipation when travelling

Site of action
• Female sexuality

• Nerves and muscles

Related remedies

Lilium tigrinum and Origanum

Sensitive type

The constitutional Platina is usually a woman, rather than a man. She is self-centred, flaunts her femininity, is always very well groomed, wearing either flashy clothes or calculatedly conservative but chic outfits. She is so fully absorbed in herself that she can only hold down a job that gives her the opportunity to be noticed or admired.

She is extremely narcissistic but puts enormous effort into making herself desirable and seductive. She has extreme mood swings.

Plumbum metallicum
Source of the remedy
The metal Lead

Suggested uses
1. Severe constipation

2. Neuralgia and muscle weakness

3. High blood pressure in subjects with atherosclerosis

Modalities
• Aggravated by movement

• Improved by firm pressure

Site of action
The central nervous system

Related remedies

Bryonia, Alumina, Causticum, Nux vomica, and Phosphorus

Podophyllum
Podophyllum in brief
Major remedy for all types of diarrhoea, as it starts

Source of the remedy
The root of the May Apple plant

Main actions
Irritation of the bowels; diarrhoea; inflammation and swelling of the right ovary

Secondary signs
Feeling of great weakness after opening the bowels. Headaches alternating with diarrhoea, and constipation alternating with diarrhoea. Thirst for large quantities of cold water. Abdominal discomfort mainly felt on the right side

Modalities
• Aggravated by hot weather, in the morning, and during teething

• Improved by lying on the abdomen

Suggested uses
1. Diarrhoea in summer and during teething: abundant, watery or with mucus, often foul smelling, and followed by a feeling of great weakness

2. Migraine alternating with diarrhoea, which generally provides relief from the pain

3. Right sided ovarian pain, with diarrhea and colic

Site of action
• The central nervous system

• The intestines

• The female reproductive system

Related remedies

China, and Arsenicum album

Prunus spinosa

Prunus spinosa in brief
Remedy for shingles around the eye and facial neuralgia

Source of the remedy
The Blackthorn plant

Main actions
Localized neuralgia or spasms, especially in the eyes, bladder, and heart

Secondary signs
Pains in the eyeball with the feeling that it will burst. Pain above the eye socket. Neuralgia in the face and teeth. All these pains make it difficult to breathe. Pain passing urine, with an urgent need to urinate

Modalities
• Aggravated by being touched and sudden movements

• Improvement at night

Suggested uses
1. Shingles

2. Facial neuralgia

3. Difficulty in passing urine, with spasms that make it impossible

Site of action
• The eye

• The immune system

• The nerves

Related remedies

Hypericum

Psorinum

Psorinum in brief
• Major nosode

• For general weakness

• Foul-smelling secretions

• Rashes and itching

Psorinum

- Allergy

- Alteration of symptoms

Source of the remedy
Nosode made from the Scabies lesions of untreated patients

Main actions
General weakness, both physical and mental; foul-smelling secretions; alternation of symptoms

Secondary signs
Extreme sensitivity to the cold, especially in summer. Raging hunger during migraines and at night. The skin is dirty, greasy, and sometimes rough. Profuse sweating after the slightest effort, foul smelling in the case of the feet. Skin rashes cause intense itching, which is aggravated by the heat of the bed and by washing.

Modalities
- Aggravated by the cold, in winter, by draughts, by contact with wool, and by the disappearance of a rash

- Improved by heat (except for the itching), by eating, in summer, by wrapping up warm, and by lying down. Feels unusually well the day before illness

Suggested uses
1. Diseases that return at regular intervals and in alternation with each other. Tendency to upper respiratory tract infections, ear infections, and recurrent bronchitis. Hay fever

2. Recurrent migraines

3. Recurrent rashes

Site of action
- The general health

- The immune system

- The skin

Sensitive type

The typical Psorinum constitutional type is a very thin person who is extremely sensitive to the cold. The skin looks dirty. The mood is pessimistic and introverted. Often depressed, these people are afraid of the future and, when they are sick, they are convinced there is no cure.

Ptelea
Source of the remedy
The bark from the root of the Hop

Main action
Liver and gall bladder problems with pain, headaches, constipation, or diarrhoea

Site of action
The liver and the gall bladder

Pulsatilla
Pulsatilla in brief
- Major remedy (polychrest)

- Catarrh

- Recurrent upper respiratory tract infections

- Varicose veins and problems with the circulation

- Problems with the digestion

Source of the remedy
The whole Pasque-flower, a type of Anemone, in flower

Main actions
Non-irritating thick, yellow discharges. Congestion of the veins, especially in the legs

Secondary signs
Constantly changing pains: 'Everything is variable with Pulsatilla'. Desire for cool air, open air, and fresh food. Aversion to hot, greasy food. Slow, difficult digestion. Abdominal bloating and belching. Diarrhoea with stools that vary greatly (no two are ever alike). Frequent colds with loss of the senses of taste and smell. Hoarseness that comes and goes. Dry cough at night, loose cough by day. Light periods that arrive late, heavier in the day than at night. Kidney pains during periods. Thick, yellow vaginal discharge. Varicose veins with stabbing pains. Purplish-red discoloration of the legs. Rashes resembling measles. Chilblains and ulcers that are purplish in colour

Modalities
• Aggravated by the heat, in a warm room, by resting, greasy foods, in puberty, in the morning, and when starting to move

• Improved by the open air, by cold applications, slow movement, consolation, and sympathy

Suggested uses
1.Digestive problems with abdominal bloating

2. Recurrent upper respiratory tract infections. Recurrent bronchitis. Bronchitis with phlegm. Ear infections

3. Period problems at puberty. Thick, yellowish vaginal discharges

4. Varicose veins, varicose ulcers, and poor circulation in the legs

5. Chilblains

Site of action
• The digestive system

• The venous system

• The reproductive system

• The ears, nose, and throat

• The emotional state

Related remedies

Ignatia, Gelsemium, Sepia, and Natrum muriaticum

Sensitive type

The Pulsatilla type is usually a very emotional woman, in search of protection and love. She is shy, depending on others because she is afraid of being alone, which she interprets as being abandoned. This hunger for affection means that, even as an adult, she allows herself to be cosseted by her mother or husband. However, in a protective environment she is able to express her potential with courage and generosity.

She looks rather fragile, is extremely sensitive to the heat, and blushes at

Pulsatilla

the slightest emotion. She likes the open air and feels uncomfortable in a room that is overheated. She is prone to problems in the venous system and often suffers with varicose veins and chilblains.

Pyrogen

Pyrogen in brief
A remedy for severe infections. It should only be used on the recommendation of a professional homeopath.

Source of the remedy
It is made from putrefied Beef

Main actions
Severe infections, with great restlessness; blood poisoning

Site of action
The immune system

Querbracho

Source of the remedy
A plant that grows in Brazil

Main actions
Respiratory problems with thick phlegm, causing a feeling of suffocation

Suggested uses
1. Excellent remedy for loosening phlegm

2. Bronchitis, particularly when chronic. Emphysema

Site of action
• The respiratory system

• The immune system

Related remedies

Hepar sulph, Silica, Kali bichromicum, and Pulsatilla.

Radium bromatum

Radium bromatum in brief
Remedy for scars and itching without a cause

Source of the remedy
Radium Bromide

Main actions
Itching all over the body; skin ulcers; low blood pressure. Bone and joint pains, especially in the spinal column

Secondary signs
Hard, thickened scars; corns; calluses; verruccas

Suggested uses
1. Violent itching with no apparent cause

2. Scars

3. Low back pain in the morning

Site of action
• The skin

• The immune system

Related remedies

Graphites and Antimonium crudum

Ranunculus bulbosus

Ranunculus bulbosus in brief
Remedy for pain in the chest wall

Source of the remedy
The whole Buttercup plant, when in flower

Rauwolfia

Main actions
Rash resembling herpes, with blisters. Acute muscular chest pains

Secondary signs
Intense, burning itching

Modalities
Aggravated by changes in the weather and temperature, by movement, and by touch, however light

Suggested uses
1. Shingles of the chest wall
2. Pain following shingles

Site of action
- The skin
- The nerves
- The immune system

Related remedies

Rhus toxicodendron, Arsenicum album, and Croton tiglium

Raphanus
Raphanus in brief
For bowel problems with wind and severe constipation, especially after an operation

Source of the remedy
The root of the Black Winter Radish.

Main actions
Excessive trapped wind in the bowel and abdominal distension

Suggested uses
1. Severe wind after an operation

2. All bowel problems involving trapped wind and severe constipation

Site of action
The bowels

Related remedies

Opium

Ratanhia
Ratanhia in brief
Good remedy for haemorrhoids and anal fissures after constipation

Source of the remedy
The root of the Ratanhia Peruviana plant

Main actions
Painful irritation of the anus and the rectum

Secondary signs
Stabbing, burning pains during and after opening the bowels. Visible, painful, burning haemorrhoids

Suggested uses
1. Constipation with pains and burning after opening the bowels

2. Haemorrhoids. Anal fissures. Inflammation of the anus and the rectum

Site of action
The blood supply of the lower bowel

Related remedies

Arnica, Aesculus, Hamamelis, Lachesis, and Nux vomica

Rauwolfia
Source of the remedy
The root of the Rauwolfia plant, which is found growing in the foothills of the Himalayas

Rauwolfia

Main actions
High blood pressure. Problems with urination and inflammation of the prostate. Loss of sexual desire and impotence in men. Depression

Site of action
• The blood vessels

• The urinary and the reproductive systems in men

Related remedies

Sulphur, Aurum metallicum, and Glonoine

Rheum palmatum
Source of the remedy
The dried root of the Rhubarb plant

Main actions
Acute diarrhoea with a sour smell, especially after eating fruit in summer, or during teething

Modalities
• Aggravated by eating acidic fruit

• Improved by bending over double and by heat

Site of action
The bowel

Related remedies

Senna, Aloe, and Chamomilla

Rhododendron
Source of the remedy
The fresh leaves of the rhododendron plant

Suggested uses
Joint pains, rheumatism and neuralgia aggravated by storms

Modalities
• Aggravated by humidity, rest, the first movement, and by fatigue

• Improved by hot, dry weather and by moving about

Site of action
The skeletal system

Related remedies

Rhus toxicodendron, Kalmia, Phosphorus, Psorinum, Sepia, and Lachesis

Rhus toxicodendron
Rhus toxicodendron in brief
Major remedy for joint pains, rashes with blisters, and influenza

Source of the remedy
The Poison Ivy plant

Main actions
Blistering of the skin. Painful stiffness and aching in the joints improved by movement. Depression

Secondary signs
Great sensitivity to cold air. Restlessness with constant need to change position. Painful furred tongue with a red triangle on the tip

Modalities
• Aggravated by rest, by rain, damp, cold weather, at night, and by lying on the painful side

• Improved by gentle movement, by changing position, and by hot, dry weather

Suggested uses
1. Joint pains following injury

2. Herpes. Shingles. Eczema

3. Influenza with joint pains

Site of action
• The joints

• The skin

• The immune system

Related remedies

Ruta, Arnica, Ranunculus bulbosus, Oscillococcinum, and Eupatorium perfoliatum

Ricinus communis
Ricinus communis in brief
Remedy for gastritis and enlargement of the breasts after giving birth

Source of the remedy
The fresh seeds of the Castor Oil plant

Main actions
Severe painless diarrhoea. Castor oil acts as a laxative, and at a low dose it stimulates milk secretion in women

Secondary signs
Pain in the stomach and liver, nausea, and vomiting

Suggested uses
1. Inflammation in the stomach (gastritis) and the intestines. Diarrhoea. Pain around the waist

2. Swelling of the breasts after giving birth

Site of action
• The digestive system

• The breasts

Robina
Robinia in brief
Minor remedy for gastric acidity

Source of the remedy
The bark of the False Acacia tree

Main actions
Pain and acidity in the stomach with regurgitation and even vomiting

Suggested uses
Digestive disorders with acidity

Site of action
The stomach

Rumex crispus
Rumex crispus in brief
Remedy for laryngitis and bronchitis

Source of the remedy
The root of the Yellow Dock plant

Main actions
Respiratory and digestive complaints. Itching while getting undressed

Secondary signs
Unrelenting, exhausting dry cough, which is triggered by breathing in cold air. Painless, urgent diarrhoea in the morning. Increased sensitivity to the cold

Modalities
• Aggravated by being uncovered, in

Rumex crispus

the evening, by breathing cold air and around 5 a.m.

- Improved by heat

Suggested uses
1. Laryngitis

2. Acute or chronic bronchitis

Site of action
The respiratory system

Related remedies

Hepar sulph, Argentum nitricum and, Calcarea fluorica

Ruta graveolens
Ruta Graveolens in brief
Remedy for traumas to the joints

Source of the remedy
The Garden Rue plant when it starts to flower

Main actions
Acts on the tendons and ligaments of the joints. Aches and bruised sensation in the joints

Secondary signs
Tired eyes after overwork

Modalities
- Aggravated by damp cold and by lying down to rest

- Improved by movement

Suggested uses
1. Fatigue, injury to the ligaments, sprains and lumbago

2. Overwork at school

Site of action
- The joints and ligaments
- The eye

Related remedies

Rhus toxicodendron and Arnica

Sabadilla
Sabadilla in brief
Remedy for hay fever

Source of the remedy
The seed of the Sabadilla Officinalis plant

Main actions
Copious, watery nasal discharge, with burning blocked nostrils. Watery eyes

Irritation in the throat, tonsillitis that spreads from left to right. Increased sense of smell

Secondary signs
Itching in the soft palate. Increased sensitivity to the scent of flowers. Vivid imagination: the slightest ailment becomes an incurable disease

Modalities
- Aggravated by the cold and at the full moon
- Improved by heat, drinks, and hot food

Suggested uses
- Hay fever
- Asthma in the pollen season

Related remedies

Allium cepa, Euphrasia, Mixed pollens and grasses

Sabal serrulata

Source of the remedy
The fresh berries of the Saw Palmetto plant

Main actions
Frequent urination at night due to an enlarged prostate. Impotence

Modalities
Aggravation at night

Site of action
The prostate and the urinary tract

Related remedies

Chimaphila and Thuja

Sabina

Source of the remedy
The young fresh tops of the branches of the Juniperus Sabina tree

Main actions
Heavy periods with pain in the lower back and pelvis

Modalities
Aggravated by heat, movement, and being touched

Site of action
The female reproductive system

Related remedies

Nitric acid, Thuja, and Cimicifuga

Salicylic acid

Source of the remedy
Salicylic Acid

Suggested uses
Vertigo with impaired hearing and ringing in the ears (Ménière's disease)

Site of action
The brain and the inner ear

Related remedies

China sulphuricum, Phosphorus, and Argentum nitricum

Sambucus nigra

Sambucus nigra in brief
Remedy for laryngitis and colds with no discharge

Source of the remedy
The flowers of the Elder-bush

Main actions
Irritation of the respiratory tract with discharge. Profuse sweating on waking up

Secondary signs
Dry cold with a completely blocked nose. Laryngitis with a harsh, troublesome cough and a feeling of suffocation. Hoarseness with thick phlegm

Modalities
Aggravation at night, with the head down, and after strong emotions

Suggested uses
1. Laryngitis

2. Dry cold

3. Whooping cough

4. Some types of asthma

Homeopathy encyclopedia

Related remedies

Rumex crispus and Hepar sulph

Sanguinaria canadensis

Sanguinaria canadensis in brief
Remedy for recurrent migraines, hot flushes in the menopause, and allergic rhinitis

Source of the remedy
The fresh root of the Bloodroot plant

Main actions
Congestion in the head, hot flushes and burning red cheeks. All the membranes become dry, burning, and irritated

Secondary signs
Migraines, especially on the right-hand side, with throbbing pain and vomiting. Catarrh with a dry, burning nose. Increased sensitivity to smells and flowers. Nasal polyps. Increased thirst

Modalities
• Aggravated by noise, light and every seven days

• Improved by sleep, darkness and passing wind

Suggested uses
1. Migraines

2. Hot flushes in the menopause

3. Hay fever

Related remedies

Lachesis, Sulphur, and Tuberculinum koch

Sarsparilla

Source of the remedy
The dried root of the Wild Liquorice plant

Main actions
Kidney colic with kidney stones, usually on the right. Dry, wrinkled skin

Modalities
Aggravated after passing urine and by damp weather

A good 'drainage remedy' for the skin and kidneys

Site of action
• The urinary tract

• The skin

Related remedies

Berberis, Pareira brava, and Calcarea carbonica

Secale cornutum

Secale cornutum in brief
Major remedy for inflamed arteries

Source of the remedy
Ergot, a fungus that is particularly common on ears of rye in damp conditions

Main actions
Violent cramps in the legs. Cold and pallor in the limbs with very intense burning feeling. The skin is very sensitive to the touch. Dry gangrene that sets in slowly

Secondary signs
Tendency to haemorrhages of dark blood. Irregular periods

Modalities
• Aggravated by heat and by being covered

• Improved by cold and by being uncovered

Suggested uses
1. Inflammations of the arteries

2. Certain types of migraine

3. Raynaud's syndrome

Site of action
• The arteries

• The female reproductive system

Related remedies

Apis mellifica and Cuprum metallicum

Selenium

Selenium in brief
Remedy for teenage acne, for hair loss, and weakness in students

Source of the remedy
The element Selenium

Main actions
Very intense physical and intellectual weakness after overworking, with general depression, and impotence without loss of sexual desire. Eczema on the palms of the hands. Acne

Secondary signs
Desire to remain lying down. Craving

for stimulants (like tea or coffee). Hair falling out

Modalities
• Aggravated by hot weather and sun, by staying up late, sexual excesses, alcoholism, and overworking

• Improved in the evenings

Suggested uses
1. Teenage acne

2 Weakness in students, due to overwork

3. Impotence with no loss of sexual desire

4. Eczema on the hands

5. Hair loss

Site of action
• The skin

• The metabolism

• The male reproductive system

Related remedies

Eugenia jambosa, China, and Kali bromatum

Senecio aureus

Source of the remedy
The whole fresh Golden Ragwort plant, when in flower

Suggested uses
Regulation of the periods

Modalities
Improved when the period arrives

Site of action
The female reproductive system

Related remedies

Pulsatilla, Natrum muriaticum, Ferrum metallicum, Calcarea phosphorica, and Tuberculinum koch

Senega
Source of the remedy
The dried root of the Snakeroot plant

Suggested uses
1. Cough with extreme difficulty in bringing up the phlegm

2. Chronic bronchitis in an elderly person

Modalities
Aggravated by the cold and in the morning

Site of action
The lungs

Related remedies

Causticum, Blatta orientalis, Antimonium tartaricum, and Carbo vegetabilis

Senna
Senna in brief
Remedy for hypoglycaemia (low blood sugar)

Source of the remedy
The dry leaflets of the Senna plant

Main actions
Digestive disorders with nausea and vomiting

Suggested uses
Low blood sugar in children, which may occur after an excessive sugar intake

Site of action
The liver

Related remedies

Lycopodium

Sepia
Sepia in brief
• Major remedy (polychrest)

• Physical exhaustion

• Disorders of the veins

• Digestive disorders

• Prolapse

• Depression

Source of the remedy
The brown 'ink' secreted by the Cuttlefish

Main actions
Sluggish circulation, especially in the pelvis and liver. Weakness of the muscles, ligaments, and walls of the veins, with varicose veins and prolapse

Secondary signs
Sensation of emptiness in the stomach with digestive disorders. A feeling of heaviness in the pelvis. Hot flushes. Constipation, as if there is an obstruction in the rectum. Haemorrhoids aggravated by walking. Yellowish-green discharges

Craving for vinegar, pickles, and acidic food. Aversion to milk and cooking smells

Modalities
• Aggravated before a storm, by cold, milk, smells, in pregnancy, and after delivery

• Improved by movement, sustained exercise, firm pressure, and heat

Suggested uses
1. Digestive disorders with constipation
2. Prolapse of the uterus
3. Haemorrhoids
4. Migraines
5. Vaginal discharge. Period problems
6. Cystitis
7. Eczema.

8. Depressive states resulting from marital difficulties

Site of action
• The central nervous system

• The emotional state

• The digestive system

• The urinary and reproductive systems

• The skin

Related remedies

Pulsatilla, Natrum carbonicum, Natrum muriaticum, and Staphysagria

Sensitive type

The constitutional Sepia is fatalistic and pessimistic, often depressed and unable

to express deep feelings. She can appear brusque, but underneath harbours tenderness and deep attachments.

She is devoted, faithful, and competent, although she may seem joyless and grumpy. She is a model employee, as long as she maintains her composure.

She is an introvert, and is slim. When illness strikes, she suffers with bloating.

Serum anguillae
Source of the remedy
Eel serum

Main actions
This remedy is very useful in cases of kidney failure. It should only be used by a professional homeopath

Site of action
The kidneys

Silica
Silica in brief
• Major remedy (polychrest)

• For recurrent infections

• Weight loss and growth problems

• After-effects of vaccinations

• Lack of self-confidence

Source of the remedy
Pure silica extracted from the Rock Crystal

Main actions
Problems with nutrition; anxiety;

chronic headaches; recurrent infections, slow to heal

Secondary signs
Increased sensitivity to the senses; weight loss and failure to thrive; great sensitivity to the cold; profuse sweating from feet and foot odour; constipation; craving for cold food; aversion to hot food and meat; upset by milk, even mother's milk

Modalities
• Aggravated by the cold, in winter, by being uncovered, by vaccinations, at the new moon, and during periods

• Improved by being warm, in summer, and by wearing warm clothes

Suggested uses
1. Weight loss in children. Problems with bone formation. Teething problems

2. Great sensitivity to the cold

3. After-effects of vaccinations

4. Osteoporosis

5. Difficulties in school. Problems with concentration. Headaches

6. Skin infections. Ear infections, sinusitis, and chronic bronchitis

Site of action
• The immune system

• The general health

• The emotional state

Related remedies

Hepar sulph and Arsenicum album

Sensitive type

The Silica type is very emotional, and remains child-like throughout their life. They are sensitive to injustice, generally frank and loyal, and they know how to be extremely sociable. However, they can be introverted, become shy, and, like all shy people, show aggression. They are anxious and unsure about everything.

As they have little confidence in their potential, they often fail to act. They do not like competition but are creative and can express themselves through art. As a result of their low energy and recurrent illnesses, they have problems in their chosen profession.

As children, they are frequently ill with infections, but gain greater resilience with age.

Solidago
Source of the remedy
The flowers of the Goldenrod plant

Main actions
Drainage of the kidneys, liver, and bladder

Site of action
The liver and the kidneys

Related remedies

Berberis

Spigelia
Spigelia in brief
• Remedy for facial neuralgia

- Palpitations

- Migraines

Source of the remedy
The entire Pinkroot plant, in bloom

Main actions
Facial neuralgia with violent stabbing or burning pains. Palpitations

Secondary signs
Migraines above the left eye, worse at night. Pain in the eyeballs

Modalities
- Aggravated at midday, by damp weather, and by storms

- Improvement when lying on the right side

Suggested uses
Left-sided migraines

Left-sided facial neuralgia

Palpitations

Site of action
- The central nervous system

- The cardiovascular system

Spongia tosta
Spongia tosta in brief
Minor remedy for laryngitis

Source of the remedy
A Sea Sponge from the Mediterranean, roasted

Main actions
Dry irritation in the nose, larynx, and trachea, with a feeling of burning and constriction. Swollen glands

Secondary signs
Waking suddenly around midnight due to difficulty breathing, with a dry, wheezy cough

Modalities
- Aggravated at night before midnight, in a warm room

- Improved by hot drinks and by eating

Suggested uses
1. Laryngitis coming on after dry cold weather

2. Whooping cough

Site of action
- The respiratory system

- The endocrine glands

Related remedies

Aconite, Rumex, and Sambucus nigra

Squilla
Source of the remedy
The bulb of the red Sea Onion plant

Main actions
Cough with watery eyes and urinary incontinence

Modalities
Aggravated by cold air and cold drinks

Site of action
The nervous system

Related remedies

Euphrasia, Natrum muriaticum, and Pulsatilla

Homeopathy encyclopedia

Stanum metallicum
Source of the remedy
The metal Tin

Suggested uses
Chronic chest problems in an exhausted person

Modalities
Aggravated by cold

Site of action
The lungs

Related remedies

Manganum, Pulsatilla, Phosphorus and, Arsenicum album

Staphylococcinum
Staphylococcinum in brief
Remedy for infections caused by the Staphylococcus bacterium

Source of the remedy
A nosode prepared from a culture of Staphylococci

Suggested uses
Infections caused by Staphylococci

Site of action
The immune system

Related remedies

Sulphur, Arsenicum album, Silica, Hepar sulph, and pyrogen

Staphysagria
Staphysagria in brief
• Major remedy (polychrest)

• For emotional setbacks or disappointments

• Intense itching

• Sexual excitement

Source of the remedy
The Delphinium plant

Main actions
Very sensitive to emotional setbacks and humiliation. Sexual excitement. Irritated skin with scabby, itchy lesions

Secondary signs
Burning sensation when not passing urine. Great hunger, especially when the stomach is full

Modalities
• Aggravated by indignation, humiliation, anger, tobacco, cuts and surgery, and from eating meat

• Improved by heat and by resting

Suggested uses
1. All emotional states following humiliation or repression of emotions, especially anger

2. Sexual obsessions

3. Cystitis in young couples

4. Prostate problems

5. Eczema on the scalp and the face, with thick scabs and violent itching

6. Styes, especially on the upper eyelid

Site of action
• The emotional state

- The nervous system

- The skin

Related remedies

Ignatia, Gelsemium, Natrum carbonicum, and Hepar sulph

Sensitive type

These people are very sensitive, easily hurt and enraged, but they cannot express their emotions because they are too inhibited or too concerned with the opinion of others. They live in a state of constant inner tension, fighting to contain their feelings. They are continually mulling over their deep feelings of hurt.

There is no particular body type characteristic of Staphysagria. These people tend to be introverted, with inscrutable faces, constantly holding their feelings in check. They suppress their anger, sinking into a state of frustration. This remedy causes a spectacular release of emotions, and thus should be used with care.

Sticta pulmonaria

Sticta pulmonaria in brief
Remedy for upper respiratory tract infections, sinusitis, and hay fever

Source of the remedy
The Lungwort plant

Main actions
Irritation of the respiratory tract. General malaise with agitation and aching

Secondary signs
The beginning of colds, before the nose starts to run, with a feeling of heaviness at the root of the nose. The nose is blocked. Constant, dry, irritating cough at night

Suggested uses
1. Dry cough that is more intense at night
2. Sinusitis
3. Hay fever, if the nose remains blocked despite sneezing

Site of action
- The respiratory system
- The immune system

Related remedies

Bryonia, Hepar sulph, Rumex crispus, and Histamine

Stramonium
Stramonium in brief
Good remedy for insomnia caused by nightmares and night terrors

Source of the remedy
Datura Stramonium, the thorn apple, when in bloom

Main actions
Violent delirium with hallucinations, incoherent rambling, and convulsions. Red congested face

Secondary signs
Night terrors with fear of the dark

Modalities
- Aggravated by darkness and by solitude

Stramonium

• Improved by soft light and by the presence of another person

Suggested uses

1. Delirium during high fevers

2. Night terrors and nightmares

Site of action

The central nervous system

Hyoscyamus

Streptococcinum

Source of the remedy

A nosode made from a culture of Streptococci bacteria, only to be used by professional homeopaths

Suggested uses

Recurrent tonsillitis and other infections caused by the Streptococcus bacterium

Site of action

The immune system

Related remedies

Hepar sulph and Pyrogen

Strontium carbonicum

Source of the remedy

The compound Strontium Carbonate

Main actions

High blood pressure; threatened strokes; neuralgia with intolerance of cold

Modalities

Improved by heat

Site of action

• The vascular system

• The nervous system

Related remedies

Sulphur, Lachesis, Aconite and Belladonna

Strophanus

Source of the remedy

The dry seed of the plant of the same name

Suggested uses

1. Disorders of the heart rhythm

2. Weak heart in elderly people, alcoholics and smokers

Modalities

Aggravated by tea, coffee and alcohol

Site of action

The cardiovascular system

Related remedies

Arsenicum album, Arsenicum iodatum, and Kali carbonicum

Sulphur

Sulphur in brief

• Major remedy (polychrest)

• Acts on Psoric conditions (see below)

• Recurrent diseases

• Allergies

• General health

• Convalescence

Source of the remedy
The element Sulphur

Main actions
Irritation of the skin with dry or moist itchy rashes. Chronic irritation of the membranes, either dry or with secretions. Congestion, especially in the liver. Localized congestion of the arteries. Problems of absorption of food.

Secondary signs
This is the remedy for what Hahnemann called Psora, which is characterized by:

• the symptoms recurring at regular intervals

• the alternation of symptoms

• the tendency to parasite infections

• a prolonged convalescence following illness

• a lack of reaction to well indicated remedies

• all these situations are indications for the use of Sulphur

Modalities
• Aggravated by heat, water, standing upright, the disappearance of a rash, excessive consumption of alcohol or sugar, and after recovering from another disease

• Improved by loss of body fluids (diarrhoea, sweating), physical exercise, sport and the open air

Suggested uses
1. Psoric complaints, particularly allergies affecting the skin: skin complaints (whatever they look like) provided they are aggravated by water and improved by cold; boils, carbuncles and styes with a tendency to recur; prolonged convalescence.

2. Problems with the circulation: hot flushes in the menopause, high blood pressure, atherosclerosis, varicose veins, and haemorrhoids.

3. Detoxification: complaints related to a sedentary lifestyle or obesity. Liver problems. Migraines

Site of action
• The general health

• The skin

• The immune system

• The heart and blood vessels

• The liver

Related remedies

Nux vomica, Gelsemium, Aurum metallicum, Psorinum, Calcarea carbonica, Arsenicum album, and Lycopodium

Sensitive type

These are active, cheerful, generous, optimistic people who love life and action. They make friends easily and are prepared to enjoy themselves with anybody who is around. They run their team, factory, or colleagues with firmness but with good humour. They are organizers or supervisors who may work in management or as company directors.

Physically speaking, there are two types of Sulphur: one is overweight, ruddy in complexion, with fleshy red lips, flared nostrils, and permanently warm skin. The other is rather thin, with thin lips and closed nostrils. The contrasting figures of Don Quixote and Sancho Panza are used to help remember these two extremes.

'Fat' Sulphur is expansive, extrovert, headstrong, and opinionated, but moved by a spirit of reconciliation and benevolence. 'Thin' Sulphur has the same qualities but with a little more restraint and a tendency for contemplation. He or she loves to talk about philosophy and metaphysics. The urge for action leads him or her away from the abstract plane, often resulting in an inventor or highly productive writer.

However, in some ways Sulphur people are fragile. Their superficial sociability can lead to excesses which affect them badly, as does the stress of even a minor ailment. It is this surprising characteristic that often leads a Sulphur person to be called a 'Colossus with feet of clay'.

Sulphur iodatum
Sulphur iodatum in brief
• Recurrent upper respiratory tract infections

• Prolonged convalescence

• Chronic eczema

• Chronic rheumatism

Source of the remedy
Sulphur Iodide

Main actions
These are influenced by the presence of Sulphur (which takes us back to the remedy Sulphur) and of iodine, which results in the swelling of the glands and the lymphatic tissues.

This remedy is not used as widely as Sulphur.

Secondary signs
Chronic swelling of the tonsils. Violent cough with copious amounts of thick phlegm

Modalities
• Aggravated by heat and exertion

• Improved by fresh air

Suggested uses
1. Recurrent upper respiratory tract infections. Tonsillitis

2. Teenage acne

3. Chronic eczema

4. Weight loss with enlarged glands

5. Chronic rheumatism

Note: Sulphur iodatum is used in preference to Sulphur in people with poor general health.

Site of action
• The immune system

• The general health

Related remedies

Arsenicum iodatum, Kali bromatum, and Hepar sulph

Sulphuric acid

Sulphuric acid in brief
Remedy for the general health in alcoholics and menopausal women and for mouth ulcers and heartburn

Source of the remedy
Diluted Sulphuric Acid

Main actions
Great weakness with trembling inside the body. Irritation of the membranes with a tendency to mouth ulcers, burning sensations in the mouth and stomach. Belching. Haemorrhages of dark blood

Secondary signs
Hot flushes in the menopause. Craving for strong drinks and fresh fruit

Modalities
• Aggravated by the strong smell of coffee

• Improved by moderate heat

Suggested uses
1. Fevers with great weakness in alcoholics and menopausal women

2. Hot flushes in the menopause

3. Mouth ulcers

4. Heartburn. Old skin ulcers

Site of action
• The immune system

• The skin and membranes

• The digestive system

Related remedies

Robinia, Amyl nitrosum, and Folliculinum

Sumbul

Source of the remedy
The root of the Musk Root plant

Main actions
Feeling of a lump in the throat when in an emotional state. Palpitations. Tendency to fainting. Unstable and anxious behaviour

Modalities
• Aggravation in the menopause, from alcohol, and from heat

• Improved by distraction

Site of action
The nervous system

Related remedies

Ignatia, Lachesis, and Iodum

Symphytum

Source of the remedy
The root of the Comphrey plant

Suggested uses
Very useful remedy to assist fracture healing

Site of action
The bones

Related remedies

Calcarea phosphorica, Ruta, Arnica, and Silica

Syphilinum
See Lueticum

Homeopathy encyclopedia

Tabacum

Tabacum in brief
Major remedy for travel sickness, also useful in treating vomiting in pregnancy and dizziness

Source of the remedy
Fresh Tobacco leaves, picked before the flowers develop

Main actions
The well-known intoxication of the first cigarette: dizziness, nausea, vomiting, low blood pressure, sweating, and diarrhoea. High blood pressure and a tendency to arterial disease. Increased secretion in the digestive and respiratory membranes, with spasms

Secondary signs
Diarrhoea, vomiting, and cold sweats

Modalities
• Aggravated by the slightest movement and by heat

• Improved by closing the eyes, in the open air, and by being fanned

Suggested uses
1. Travel sickness (car, boat, aeroplane, etc.)

2. Vomiting in pregnancy

3. Ménière's disease (dizziness, ringing in the ear, and impaired hearing). Vertigo in people with atherosclerosis

Site of action
• The central nervous system

• The inner ear

Related remedies
Cocculus

Taraxacum

Source of the remedy
The dandelion, whole, and in flower

Main actions
Liver disorders. Jaundice. Painful, dirty tongue, with blotches (geographical tongue)

This remedy is a good liver 'drainage remedy'

Site of action
The liver

Related remedies

Hydrastis, Lycopodium, Carduus marianus, Phosphorus, China, and Natrum Muriaticum

Tarentula hispanica

Tarentula in brief
Good remedy for behavioural problems in children

Source of the remedy
The whole Lycosa Tarentula spider

Main actions
Muscular, psychological, and sexual excitement, increased sensory perception

Secondary signs
Extremely changeable behaviour, varying from great exuberance to profound sadness. Violent, incoherent delirium.

Constant restlessness. Intense headaches

Modalities
• Aggravated by grief, cold, damp weather, and all sensory stimuli

• Improved by music and the open air in mild weather

Suggested uses
1. Behavioural problems, with restlessness and spasms, especially in children

2. Inconsistent school results

3. Sexual excitement

Site of action
• The central nervous system

• The emotional state

Related remedies

Lachesis

Tellurium
Source of the remedy
The metal Tellurium

Suggested uses
1. Chronic sciatica

2. Chronic ear infection with discharge

Modalities
Aggravated by being touched and jolted

Site of action
• The bones and ligaments

• The ear

Related remedies

Hepar sulph

Terebinthina
Source of the remedy
Turpentine, made from the resin of the Larch

Main actions
Blood in the urine, originating from the bladder or kidneys

Site of action
The urinary system

Related remedies

Thuja, Phosphorus, Cantharis, Mercurius corrosivus, Eel serum, and Arsenicum album

Teucrium marum
Source of the remedy
The Cat Thyme plant, in flower

Main actions
Polyps in the nose; allergic rhinitis; itching in the anus and rectum

Site of action
• The nose

• The rectum

Related remedies

Thuja, Nitric acid, and Silica

Thallium
Source of the remedy
The element Thallium

Main actions
Alopecia (hair loss), whether widespread or in a limited area

Thallium

Site of action
The scalp

Related remedies

Graphites, Sepia, Thuja, Sulphur, Natrum muriaticum, and Silica

Theridion
Source of the remedy
The whole Orange-back spider

Main actions
Increased sensitivity with great intolerance to the slightest noise

Modalities
Aggravated by travelling, by all stimuli and by closing the eyes

Site of action
The central nervous system

Related remedies

Asarum, Nux vomica, Lachesis, and Lycopodium

Thlaspi bursa pastoris
Source of the remedy
The Shepherd's Purse whole, when in flower

Suggested uses
Heavy periods

Site of action
The female reproductive system

Related remedies

Calcarea carbonica, Arnica, and Hamamelis

Thuja occidentalis
Thuja occidentalis in brief
- Major remedy (polychrest)
- For sycosis
- Ill effects of vaccinations
- Ill effects of allopathic treatments
- Skin complaints
- Polyps and tumours
- Prostate hypertrophy
- Reduction in intellectual sharpness

Source of the remedy
The leafy branches of the White Cedar

Main actions
Eruptions: papules, blisters, and pustules. Warts and other growths. Swelling of the glands, the tonsils, and the spleen. Neuralgia. Nervousness, anxiety, and a tendency to obsessions

Secondary signs
This is the main remedy for what Hahnemann called Sycosis, characterized by:

- chronic fluid retention

- chronic discharges

- the production of small tumours on the skin

- slow, insidious, and progressive development

Modalities
- Aggravated by the cold damp, wind, tea, coffee, greasy food, vaccinations, and allopathic medicines

• Improved by stretching

Suggested uses
1. All sycotic conditions, particularly the ill effects of vaccinations and allopathic treatments, obesity, and chronic rheumatism

2. Warts. Skin complaints. Blemishes on the nails. Hair loss

3. Neuralgia. Obsessions

4. Discharges that continue after urethritis. Prostate hypertrophy. Polyps. Urinary infection. Fibroids

Site of action
The immune system

The general health

The skin

The emotional state

Related remedies

Thuja is one of the most widely used remedies in homeopathy and it can be used with a very large number of other medicines.

Sensitive type

These are pessimists who are ill at ease and never stop trying to explain their bad luck. They are never cheerful and confident, and are constantly sad, which prevents them from making any commitment to an active life. This condition is acquired gradually and is more common in middle age.

They think and work in slow motion,

held back by their fears. Their obsessive side, however, can make them efficient in jobs requiring precision. They like to see work well done and are diligent in the tasks they undertake.

Thuja is usually a sturdy person, somewhat fat, especially in the trunk, but with rather thin legs. Their skin is greasy and they suffer with cellulite. Their nails are often striated and prone to breaking. When Thuja is thinner he or she is more lively, both physically and mentally, and tries to overcompensate for the inner fears and torment.

Trillium

Trillium in brief
Minor remedy for heavy periods caused by fibroids

Source of the remedy
The rhizome of the Birthroot plant

Main actions
Haemorrhages, especially from the uterus, with bright red blood and a tendency to fainting. Painful, very heavy periods, coming every two weeks

Suggested uses
1. Heavy bleeding from fibroids
2. Problems in the menopause
3. Period problems with a tendency to fainting

Site of action
The female reproductive system

Related remedies

Sabina and Secale cornutum

Tuberculinum aviare

Source of the remedy
This nosode is prepared from Tubercular Hens. It is more gentle than Tuberculinum koch

Suggested uses
Chronic infections in children: recurrent ear, nose, and throat infections, chest infections and recurrent asthma

Site of action
The immune system

Related remedies

Hepar sulph and Silica

Tuberculinum koch

Tuberculinum koch in brief
• A major nosode

• For weight loss

• Recurrent ear, nose, and throat infections

• Colitis

• Nervous complaints

• Recurrent migraines

Source of the remedy
This nosode is prepared from Human Tubercular matter

Main actions
Rapid reduction in weight, leading to weakness and emotional fragility. Extreme sensitivity to cold. Discharges from the whole respiratory tract and recurrent infections. Dry or wet eczema with intense itching aggravated by the warmth of the bed and improved by cold water

Secondary signs
Excessive sweating at the slightest exertion. Nocturnal coughing. Diarrhoea around 5 a.m. Aversion to meat and craving for cold milk

Modalities
• Aggravated by the slightest physical exertion, in a closed room, by standing up, changes in the weather, the heat of the bed, the cold damp, and on waking up in the morning

• Improved in the fresh air, by resting, and by travelling

Suggested uses
1. Weight loss with no reduction in appetite

2. Rickets in children

3. Recurrent respiratory tract and ear, nose, and throat infections

4. Digestive problems with colitis, affecting the general health

5. Regularly recurring conditions: migraines, cystitis, boils, and styes

Site of action
• The immune system

• The central nervous system

• The emotional state

Sensitive type

The Tubercular type remains thin, despite a hearty appetite. He, or she, is irritable and quick to anger. He or she tires easily and easily becomes pessimistic and disillusioned with life.

Tuberculinum residuum

Tuberculinum residuum in brief
Minor remedy, used for scar tissue, adult acne, and prostate enlargement

Source of the remedy
A nosode prepared from the filtered products of Tuberculosis

Main actions
Arthritis with stiffening and deformities. Scarred tissues

Suggested uses
1. Scars, especially keloid scars

2. Enlargement of the prostate

3. Severe acne on the shoulders and back

Site of action
• The general health

• The skin

• The prostate

Related remedies

Graphites and Thuja

Uric acid

Uric acid in brief
Minor remedy for gout and high levels of uric acid

Source of the remedy
Uric acid

Suggested uses
1. Kidney stones made of uric acid

2. Gout

Urtica urens

Urtica urens in brief
Remedy for urticaria

Source of the remedy
The stinging nettle used whole

Main actions
Stinging, burning swellings with unbearable itching

Secondary signs
Urticaria with stinging and burning

Modalities
Aggravated by cold water

Suggested uses
Urticaria

Site of action
• The immune system

• The skin

Related remedies

Apis mellifica and Histamine

Ustilago

Source of the remedy
The parasitic fungus found on corn, known as Corn Smut

Main actions
Bleeding from the uterus and the cervix. This remedy can be useful, as a complement to orthodox treatment, after delivery or an abortion

Site of action
The female reproductive system

Related remedies

Sulphur and Lachesis

Valeriana

Source of the remedy
The fresh root of the Valerian plant

Main actions
Nervousness with increased sensitivity. Restlessness. Violent pains with spasms and cramps

Modalities
• Aggravated by the slightest setback and by the least pain

• Improved by movement

Site of action
The central nervous system

Related remedies

Ignatia, Cuprum metallicum, and Chamomilla

Veratrum album

Veratrum album in brief
Major remedy for severe diarrhoea

Source of the remedy
The root of the White Hellebore plant

Main actions
Sever gastro-enteritis resembling cholera: copious amounts of diarrhoea and vomiting with profuse sweating. Collapse and cramps in the bowels. General weakness, to the point of exhaustion. The whole body feels cold, but there is internal burning

Secondary signs
Aggravated by cold, damp weather. Improved by heat

Suggested uses
Severe diarrhoea, with cramping pains, severe weakness, and profuse sweating

Site of action
• The bowels

• The immune system

Related remedies

Arsenicum album

Veratrum viride

Veratrum viride in brief
Minor complementary remedy for subjects with high blood pressure, and after sunstroke

Source of the remedy
The root of the American White Hellebore

Main actions
Congested red face with headache, throbbing in the arteries in the neck, and restless delirium

Suggested uses
1. Congestion in people with high blood pressure, who are obese and big eaters

2. Sunstroke

Site of action
The cardiovascular system

Related remedies

Apis mellifica and Belladonna

Verbascum

Source of the remedy
The whole Mullein, when in bloom

Main actions
Facial neuralgia that recurs at regular intervals. Nasal discharge and laryngitis with burning discharge

Modalities
Aggravated by any movement, by being touched, pressure, or a draught of air

Site of action
The central nervous system

Related remedies

Cedron, Bryonia, and Kali iodatum

Viburnum opulus

Viburnum opulus in brief
Minor remedy for period problems

Source of the remedy
The bark of Cramp Elder tree

Main actions
Congestion and painful spasms in the female reproductive system. Late, light and short periods

Secondary signs
Sudden cramping pains that spread into the thighs and back

Modalities
• Aggravated by jolting

• Improved by resting and pressure

Suggested uses
Problems related to light periods with cramps and a tendency to faint

Site of action
The female reproductive system

Related remedies

Caulophyllum, Colocynthis, and Magnesia phosphorica

Vinca minor

Source of the remedy
The whole Lesser Periwinkle, in flower

Main actions
Great fatigue, exhaustion with prostration, and trembling. Haemorrhages

Site of action
The general health

Related remedies

Phosphorus and Carbo vegetabilis

Viola odorata

Source of the remedy
The whole Sweet-scented violet, when in bloom

Main actions
Rheumatic pains in the small joints, especially the wrists

Site of action
The skeletal system

Viola tricolor

Source of the remedy
The Wild Pansy, in bloom

Main actions
Weeping infected eczema on the scalp. Impetigo with thick yellow scabs

Site of action
The skin

Vipera berus

Vipera in brief
Major remedy for disorders of the veins

Source of the remedy
The venom of the Common Viper

Main actions
Haemorrhage and bruising. Inflammations of veins and lymphatic vessels. Phlebitis

Suggested uses
1. Phlebitis
2. Varicose veins

Site of action
The veins

Related remedies

Lachesis

Xanthoxylum fraxineum

Source of the remedy
The bark of the Prickly Ash sapling

Suggested uses
1. Neuralgia with increase in body weight
2. Pains in the left ovary

Modalities
Aggravation on the left side

Site of action
• The nerves
• The female reproductive system

Related remedies

Mezereum, Platina, and Chamomilla

Zea italica

Source of the remedy
Corn-silk

Suggested uses
1. Dry, scaly eczema
2. Psoriasis
3. This is a drainage remedy for the skin

Site of action
The skin

Related remedies

Berberis and Saponaria

Zincum metallicum

Zincum metallicum in brief
Minor remedy for overwork at school and problems with mobility

Source of the remedy
The metal zinc

Main actions
Mental exhaustion with restlessness. Slowness in thought and formulation of ideas

Secondary signs
Continuous movements of feet and legs

Suggested uses
1. Inability to 'sit still'
2. Intellectual fatigue and overwork at school
3. Intolerance of wine and other types of alcohol

Site of action
• The central nervous system
• The nerves

Related remedies

Kali carbonicum and manganum

Homeopathy encyclopedia

Homeopathy encyclopedia

Homeopathy encyclopedia

Your own notes

Homeopathy encyclopedia

Homeopathy encyclopedia

Homeopathy encyclopedia

Homeopathy encyclopedia